Understanding Children's Drawings

Understanding Children's Drawings

CATHY A. MALCHIODI

Foreword by Eliana Gil

THE GUILFORD PRESS
New York   London

Published by The Guilford Press
A Division of Guilford Publications, Inc.
72 Spring Street, New York, NY 10012
http://www.guilford.com

Printed in the United States of America

This book is printed on acid-free paper.

Last digit is print number: 9 8 7 6 5 4 3 2 1

Library of Congress Cataloging-in-Publication Data

Malchiodi, Cathy A.
    Understanding children's drawings / Cathy A. Malchiodi.
      p. cm.
    Includes bibliographical references and index.
    ISBN 1-57230-351-4 (hc.). — ISBN 1-57230-372-7 (pbk.)
    1. Children's drawings—Psychological aspects. 2. Art therapy for
children. 3. Brief psychotherapy. I. Title.
AJ505.A7M353 1998
155.4—dc21

                                      98-17311
                                         CIP

To Rawley Silver and Jimmy Santiago Baca
in admiration of their work with children through art

Foreword

Cassie, a 6-year-old child who worried about her mother's drug abuse, drew a picture of a cave with bats hanging on the cave walls. She was quite artistic and the "life of the picture" was grim and foreboding. Such was the child's externalization of nighttime fears about the dangerous environment in which her mother lived.

When I asked Cassie to tell me about the cave and the bats who lived in it, she seemed surprised. Her previous therapist did not know how to talk with Cassie about her drawings and had missed some valuable clues that could have been helpful in understanding what Cassie was trying to communicate in her art. In exploring Cassie's drawing with her, and in speaking with her grandmother, I found out that Cassie's bats were very real to her. Her grandmother confided that, in a drug-induced state, Cassie's mother swatted away imaginary bats. Through her drawing, Cassie was conveying not only her mother's hallucination, but also her wish to be heard and understood through her art.

A wide variety of therapists who work with children, including myself, stock our therapy rooms with toys, art materials, sandtrays, and miniatures. When we do so we invite our child clients to engage with these materials. This invitation is an awesome opportunity to facilitate, enhance, and promote the child's therapy. Yet clinicians may not take full advantage of what they can learn from children's art. My own professional curiosity, education, and experience of children's artwork has evolved over time. I look back and feel mortified about clients I did not see or hear as perceptively as I might have. I can't tell you how many times I've said to myself, "If only I'd known then what I know now. . . ."

Understanding clients' art expressions is an important clinical skill. It involves learning how to introduce art in therapy, how to think about it, and how to respond. As my skill level increases, my perception of art and its value in therapy is transformed, and my respect for the process, the power, and the potential of therapeutic art deepens.

And this brings me to the reason I'm writing this foreword. Cathy Malchiodi is one of the foremost art therapists in the country. She is one of the most respected theorists and practitioners, with an active involvement in all phases of the current evolution of art therapy as a distinct field of study. I studied her work long before I met her, and she has been a constant source of wonder to me. Her first book, *Breaking the Silence: Art Therapy with Children from Violent Homes,* chronicled the experience of children who lived with their mothers at battered women's shelters. That book changed my perception of the value of children's artwork and its uses in therapy.

This new volume is a thorough, inspired, and scholarly work which I savored in my first reading and which will prove invaluable in rereading. Malchiodi utilizes her vast background as an art educator and therapist to bring to the surface substantive knowledge combined with rich clinical experience. The end product is an accessible, informative, ethical book filled with practical suggestions of "what to do," with clear guidelines for approaching the work with sensitivity and care.

Malchiodi documents the broad utilization of both the process and the content of art in therapy as a vehicle for the child to accomplish many things: to express feelings, thoughts, and perceptions; to communicate through symbols and visual narratives; to provide relief from distressing emotions; to work through trauma and loss; to express somatic concerns; and to encourage interaction with the therapist. At the same time, drawings provide the therapist with a nonthreatening tool in enhancing communication; they can assist the therapist in evaluating growth and development; help in understanding children's perceptions of self and family; and aid in the assessment of trauma, emotional difficulties, and interpersonal problems.

In this book, children are seen in their full complexity: what they draw and the way they draw are not simply reflections of the child's needs, wishes, and fears, but are strongly influenced by other factors such as the child's stage of development, sociocultural influences, and the context in which the child is drawing. Malchiodi puts aside assumptions that a drawing could have a fixed meaning and guides and challenges the therapist to address the multidimensional aspects of children's drawings and to respect the uniqueness of each child's artwork.

I am so enthusiastic about the wisdom in the following pages that I want to end this foreword so you can start on your learning journey. At last there is a single source that synthesizes the vast database gleaned from empirical and clinical sources.

This book will greatly enhance your understanding of children's drawings created in therapy. At the same time, it will fortify and stretch your perceptions, insights, and competence level by giving you a firm knowledge base, clear guidelines and directions, and a solid foundation in theory and practice.

ELIANA GIL, PHD
Starbright Training Institute
for Child and Family Play Therapy
Rockville, MD

Acknowledgments

If it takes a village to raise a child, then it certainly takes one to write a book on children's drawings. I would like to thank the following people who helped to make *Understanding Children's Drawings* possible: First and foremost, Susan Spaniol for reading the initial manuscript while it was still in its early stages, finding its strengths and weaknesses, and providing insightful feedback; Nancy Boyd Webb for sharing practical advice that helped to shape this text and make its contents "user friendly" for all professionals who work with children; Carol Thayer Cox and Lori Vance for their generosity as friends and colleagues; Ian Vance-Curzan for drawings and cover art; Rawley Silver and David Henley for lending illustrations; and Eliana Gil for graciously writing the Foreword.

Special thanks go to Rochelle Serwator for providing meticulous editorial advice, crafting sentences, and seeing me through revisions. Her suggestions and guidance were not only invaluable to the development of this book, but also immensely helpful to my continuing growth as a writer.

Finally, my gratitude goes to the children whose creative expressions have stimulated my thinking, enriched my clinical work, and made this book a reality.

Preface

Throughout my experience as an art educator, art therapist, and clinical counselor, understanding children's art has been a process of personal evolution. In all my encounters with children, I have been repeatedly fascinated and surprised by what they communicate through their drawings and have learned a great deal about them through their art expressions. As a result of these fortunate encounters, I discovered that drawings offer therapists a potent tool for understanding children's thoughts, feelings, fantasies, conflicts, and worries, as well as perceptions and reflections of the world around them.

In writing this book, I have had the chance to recall the many experiences I have had with children that have shaped my philosophy on their drawings. One of my earliest experiences was in a small summer recreation program in my home town in Connecticut where I developed a relationship with a shy and withdrawn 8-year-old girl. In retrospect, I realize that the girl probably was depressed, came from a troubled home, and possibly had other emotional problems. However, what I remember most vividly was her joy and comfort in spending afternoons drawing with me. It seemed that, although her behavior and demeanor were often misunderstood by other children and the recreation staff, she spoke poignantly about herself through her drawings, depicting what she could not verbalize because of depression, fear, and lack of self-esteem. I think she realized that I understood her through her drawings and that I accepted what she told me about herself through her pictures. In essence, we had found a common ground where we could relate to each other with safety and mutual respect.

After that experience, I went on to train as an artist and eventually as an art educator, a natural outcome of the interest I had developed in working with children that summer. I became interested in art not only because of my experiences with children but also because I felt it was an authentic way to express myself, both as a child and as an adult. Like many artists, I have often utilized art to understand and make sense of trauma in my own life. Art expression has been the key to my understanding of personal loss, crisis, and emotional upheaval when words could not adequately express or contain meaning.

My work as an art educator after college involved teaching art in private elementary schools with young children and later with adolescents in public high schools. Some of these children and adolescents were gifted, some were just plain "normal," and some had physical, developmental, or emotional problems. As an art teacher, I had the opportunity to interact with hundreds of children and to realize that, for children, drawing is representative of many things—development, personality, emotions, interpersonal relationships, and cultural and societal influences.

One adolescent boy in particular, a student in a public school art class, profoundly enhanced my thinking about art expression. Through his drawings and paintings, he gradually began to share with me his rage toward his abusive parents, his despair over his home situation, and his own feelings of self-destruction. Although not trained in psychology or art therapy at that time, I recognized that the art he shared with me revealed his desperation and thoughts of suicide. It was through his artwork that he helped me to understand his emotional pain and depression and permitted me to intervene on his behalf before he carried out his plans to take his own life. From this experience and others with children and adolescents, I learned about the power that visual images have to express the most painful and unspoken parts of the self and how these nonverbal messages can be, in some cases, life saving.

My work with adolescents led me to become more interested in the psychological aspects of art, taking me back to graduate school to train as an art therapist. My graduate training in art therapy changed my career course to more clinically related work with both children and adolescents, in hospitals, shelters, and schools. My first job after graduation was as an art therapist at a shelter for battered women and their children, most of whom were traumatized by domestic violence, and often physical and sexual abuse. From these children, I learned how the impact of trauma can be expressed through art, and, for many children who have been abused or are witnesses to violence, I learned that art is one of the only ways to communicate their experiences and crises. Compelling depictions of depression, anxiety, fear, and loneliness came forth in their drawings, demonstrating the power of art both to reflect and contain emotions when words were not possible.

I later worked in hospitals with children with various cancers, renal diseases, trauma such as burns or accidents, and orthopedic problems. In addition to the profound emotional problems with which these children struggled, aspects of their somatic conditions emerged in their art. Another element also became apparent in their drawings: the spiritual issues that children who are threatened with serious illness or life-threatening conditions face. Drawing for these children became a place to express not only crisis and loss, but also their feelings and perceptions about God, heaven, death, and dying.

Today, in my work as a therapist, supervisor, and consultant, it is exciting to see that many helping professionals who work with children are aware of the unique potential of drawings in therapy. Children's drawings have captivated not only those who love the charm and naiveté of children's art but also psychologists, psychiatrists, counselors, play therapists, social workers, and other mental health professionals who have recognized the applications of children's art expressions in assessment and treatment. Many helping professionals are curious about how to decipher children's drawings and how to begin to understand their possible meanings. More importantly, those who work with children realize that drawing is a child-appropriate form of communication, that it allows a level of comfort and a sense of safety sometimes not found through talk therapy alone, and can provide an alternative way of interacting with children in treatment. With the advent of brief forms of therapy and the increasing pressures to complete treatment in a limited number of sessions, therapists increasingly find that drawing helps children to communicate relevant issues and problems quickly, thus expediting assessment and intervention.

THE PURPOSE OF THIS BOOK

The purpose of this book is two-fold. First and foremost, it is to provide an overview of *the multidimensional aspects of children's drawings.* Numerous books and articles have been published over the last several decades on the use of drawings for the purpose of evaluation and therapy. Although there is a great deal of material describing the use of children's drawings, it is difficult for therapists who simply want a broad overview of children's drawings to obtain the information they need easily.

In addressing the need for a basic text on children's drawings, I have integrated my own experiences with historical and contemporary research, distilling this material into practical information for therapists who want to enhance their understanding of children through their drawings. In addition to information on the variety of meanings of children's drawings, special attention has been given to explaining drawings from different perspectives (developmental, emotional content, interpersonal, somatic, and spiritual) and the importance of contextual influences. Although my primary training is as an art therapist, this book is intended to be a handbook for the wide continuum of mental health professionals who work with children, and it is written with psychologists, counselors, social workers, and play therapists in mind.

The second aspect of the book's intent is to help therapists consider *ways of working with children and their drawings*. In therapeutic work with children, drawing can quickly bring to the surface issues that are relevant to treatment, thereby improving the therapist's ability to intervene and assist troubled children. The book provides practical guidelines about how to assist children in the process of drawing, what questions to ask and when to ask them, and how to help children who are resistant to drawing. The process of drawing and the therapist's role in the process are seen as integral parts of understanding children and their drawings.

This book emphasizes both understanding the phenomenology of children's art expressions and acknowledging these expressions as complex reflections of many factors and influences. If therapists are able to put aside the notion that drawings only have specific diagnostic uses in therapy or that images have singular meanings, they have many ways to respond and help children through drawings made in therapy. By approaching children's drawings from the multidimensional perspectives described in this book, therapists will naturally learn more about children's experiences and be more informed about their problems and potential.

There is one central message interwoven throughout this book: Offering children the opportunity to communicate through drawing is a strategy that can easily be a part of every therapist's repertoire. Most therapists, at least when they were young children, have had the experience of drawing, and as adults are familiar with typical materials such as pencils, crayons, and felt marking pens used in drawing. Also, for the professional who wishes to use therapeutic art activities with children, drawing is the most easily available and one of the simpler media with which to begin. Although other modalities can help children express themselves, drawing is certainly one of the most economical, while still offering a wide range of expressive possibilities.

Finally, although understanding what children are communicating through their drawings is the major thrust of this book, acknowledging the potent process that is involved in drawing is also recognized. I believe that therapists who work with children not only are intrigued with what children's drawings say about them but also are interested in how drawing itself can be of help to the children they see in therapy. While it is true that art can provide a window to children's problems, traumatic memories, and other powerful and troublesome experiences, its primary purpose is to give the child another language with which to share feelings, ideas, perceptions, fantasies, and observations about self, others, and the environment. By accepting and respecting the multidimensional aspects of children's art expressions, therapists can facilitate children's explorations of thoughts, feelings, and ideas and can provide a way for both child and therapist to communicate through images rather than words alone. In this way, drawings can serve as a catalyst for increased interaction and interchange, thus expanding the effectiveness and depth of the relationship between therapist and child.

Contents

A Historical Perspective on Children's Drawings

There has been a growing fascination over the past century with the emotional and psychological aspects of children's art expressions, particularly from the fields of psychology, psychiatry, and art therapy. Drawing has been undeniably recognized as one of the most important ways that children express themselves and has been repeatedly linked to the expression of personality and emotions. Children's drawings are thought to reflect their inner worlds, depicting various feelings and relating information concerning psychological status and interpersonal style. Although children may use drawing to explore, to problem solve, or simply to give visual form to ideas and observations, the overall consensus is that art expressions are uniquely personal statements that have elements of both conscious and unconscious meaning in them and can be representative of many different aspects of the children who create them.

Most therapists who work with children recognize that drawing is an effective therapeutic modality because it may help children express themselves in ways that language cannot. However, because drawing is such a common and natural approach in work with children, many therapists may think that the use of art expression in the assessment and evaluation of children is simply a normal extension of their play activities and are unfamiliar with the extensive history of investigations of children's art expressions. The study of children's drawings actually has quite a long tradition in the fields of psychiatry, psychology, art therapy, and education. This long-standing fascination with children's art has generated a great deal of information on how children use drawing to express themselves, information that clinicians, counselors, and teachers who use drawings with children should know.

This chapter briefly reviews the various ways that children's drawings have been studied, investigated, and examined over the last 100 years. In using drawings as part of assessment, intervention, or treatment, it is first important for therapists to appreciate how the history of clinical applications and projective drawing tests as well as more recent developments have impacted understanding of the developmental, cognitive, and psychological aspects of children's drawings. All of these viewpoints can provide the professional who uses drawings in therapy with children with a more complete foundation for responding to the form, style, and content of children's art expressions, a more accurate and complete perception of children, and can greatly enhance and inform the use of drawings with children in treatment.

PROJECTIVE TESTS: DRAWINGS AS MEASURES OF INTELLIGENCE AND PERSONALITY

For more than a hundred years, there has been an attraction to connecting art expressions with the personalities of their creators. In the late 1800s and early 1900s, interest grew in Europe in the art of mentally ill, institutionalized adults, and many noted that drawings by patients could be used as aids in diagnosis of psychopathology (MacGregor, 1989). Most writers of this time period believed that the art expressions of mentally ill patients confirmed their diagnoses, particularly schizophrenia. For example, Tardieu's (1872) Etude Médico-Légale sur la Folie included reproductions of patients' drawings providing criteria for a legally acceptable diagnosis of mental illness. Simon (1876) published an article "L'Imagination dans la Folie" ("Imagination and Madness") which included a series of studies of drawings by the mentally ill. Lombroso (1895) also observed that drawings and paintings of the mentally ill provided insight into the psychological state of these individuals.

During the 1920s, Hans Prinzhorn, an art historian turned psychiatrist, began soliciting art created by mental patients from other doctors and hospitals throughout Europe. He collected 5,000 artworks by over 500 patients, works that would later become the basis of the publication Artistry of the Mentally Ill (1972). This collection drew attention to the notion that art expressions might have both diagnostic value as well as play an important role in rehabilitation (MacGregor, 1989).

The forefathers of modern psychology, Freud and Jung, both had interests in the interconnections among art, symbols, and personality. Freud observed that images represented forgotten or repressed memories and that these symbols were likely to emerge through either dreams or art expressions. He wrote about the images presented in dreams and reported that his patients frequently said that they could draw their dreams, but they were unable to describe them in words. Freud also believed that universal human conflicts and neuroses motivated artists to artistic creation. This observation inspired and eventually confirmed the belief that art expression could be a route to understanding the inner world of the human psyche.

Jung saw images in a different way, placing importance on them in terms of more universal meanings. Jung was particularly interested in psychological content of art expressions, including his own drawings and those of his patients. Unlike Freud who never asked his patients to draw their dream images, Jung often encouraged patients to draw. "To paint what we see before us," he said, "is a different art from painting what we see within" (1954; p. 47). Jung understood the important connections between image and psyche, and he developed a foundation for understanding symbolic meanings in imagery through his studies of archetypes and universalities inherent in visual art. Fantasy through symbol production was thought by Jung to be the psyche's attempt to evolve and, in cases of trauma or distress, a way to heal oneself (Jung, 1956).

Although there has probably always been a fascination with children's drawings, formal exploration of children's art came out of the growing interest in the art of people with mental illness at the turn of the century and the increasing prominence of the work of both Freud and Jung. Attention to children's drawings paralleled both the attraction to art created by mental patients and the development of child psychology at that time. Initial studies of children's art expression centered around observing both what children drew and how they drew at different ages. Children's drawings were the subject of an early study by Cooke (1885) who wrote an article describing stages of artistic development and emphasizing the importance of this finding for children's education. Ricci (1887) also published his observations on the drawings of Italian children, possibly the earliest collection of children's drawings on record (Harris, 1963). During the late 1800s and early 20th century, there were many descriptions of the developmental levels in children's artistic expression discussing various stages that children go through in their artistic behavior. (Harris has written a comprehensive historical review of these very early studies of children's drawings; see Chapter 4 for more information on the developmental stages of children's art expression.)

Early research on children's drawings began with an emphasis on their use in determining intelligence level. Burt (1921) used a drawing of a man as one of several intelligence tests and concluded that the drawing showed less relationship to a child's intellectual abilities than tests of reading, mathematical, or writing skills. However, he did see the advantage of drawings with children since they were less dependent on learned skills such as arithmetic or writing. Goodenough (1926) and later Harris (1963) explored age norms for human figure drawings, relating drawings to mental age rather than chronological age.

Goodenough (1926) developed what she referred to as the Draw-A-Man (DAM) test, based on the assumption that certain aspects of drawing performance correlate to a child's mental age and therefore could be used as a measure of intelligence. The subject of a man was chosen because of its universality and preference among children, as opposed to a drawing of a house, which was thought to have more variability across cultures. Goodenough considered the number of details, correct proportions between body parts, and motor coordination as demonstrated by the fluency of lines and integration of parts.

Goodenough also observed that the DAM test revealed personality traits in addition to intelligence; this supposition was later defended by the work of Buck (1948), Machover (1949), and others. In work with children, the human figure drawing continued to be popular and the subject of many projective drawing studies during the first half of the 20th century. The intuitive consensus became that children's drawings of humans provide important information about themselves and about their perceptions of other people. In addition to the use of children's drawings of human figures in assessment of intelligence (Burt, 1921; Goodenough, 1926; Harris, 1963), other theorists and researchers began to look at children's drawings as indicative of development (Koppitz, 1968) and personality characteristics (Koppitz, 1968; Machover, 1949; Hammer, 1958).

Emergence of Projective Drawing Tests

Around 1940, the idea that drawings could be used to determine emotional aspects and personality began to take hold, and drawings were studied as visual representations of internal psychological states. The term "projective drawing" emerged and projective drawing tests were developed, based on the accepted belief that drawings represent the inner psychological realities and the subjective experiences of the person who creates the images. Projective techniques include not only drawings, but also include devices such as sentence completion tests, picture tests such as the Rorschach and the Thematic Apperception Test (TAT), and word association tests.

Projective drawing tests were based on the idea that children's responses through drawing specific figures such as people or common themes such as houses, trees and figures, would reflect personality, perceptions, and attitudes. Drawing was thought to offer an alternative to self-expression that could bring out information about children that words alone could not. As the belief that drawings could be projective took hold, various projective drawing tasks for the purpose of assessing personality increasingly appeared in psychological and psychiatric literature; between 1940 and 1955, there was an abundance of published research on their use (see *Journal of Projective Techniques* and *Journal of Clinical Psychology* during this time period).

One of the more well-known projective drawing tests is Buck's (1948, 1966) House–Tree–Person (HTP), created as an ancillary to intelligence tests that were being developed during the same time. Three objects (a house, a tree, and a person) were selected because of their familiarity to even very young children and their ability to stimulate associations and projective material. Buck asserted that the HTP encouraged conscious and unconscious associations; for example, the house drawing was throught to bring out information on issues related to the home and those living in the home, while the tree drawing was thought to be representative of the child's psychological development and feelings about the environment. Evaluations of house, tree, and person drawings were based on the presence or absence of features, details, proportions, and perspective, and use of color, as a chromatic set of drawings may be requested as part of the protocol. A questionnaire also was part of the evaluation procedure.

Of all the projective drawing tests of the time period, Machover's (1949) Draw-A-Person projective test and work on personal projection in human figure drawings seems to be the most widely known, becoming a major influence on almost all research on clinical applications of human figure drawings, including children's. Despite the problematic aspects and assumptions of Machover's work (Golomb,

1990), it still is referenced by many clinicians and researchers (Drach-nik, 1995; Hammer, 1958,1997; Jolles, 1971; Cantlay, 1996; Mitchell & McArthur, 1994; Oster & Montgomery, 1996; Wohl & Kaufman, 1985). Her conceptual framework, firmly rooted in psychoanalytic thought, is based on the following belief: "the human figure drawn by an individual who is directed to 'draw a person' relates intimately to the impulses, anxieties, conflicts, and compensation characteristic of that individual. In some sense, the figure drawn is the person, and the paper corresponds to the environment" (p. 35).

It is apparent from this description that Machover presumed drawings, particularly those of human figures, to be representative of conflictual aspects, defense mechanisms, neuroses, and pathology of their creators. She attached specific symbolic meanings to parts of the human figure and other details in drawings, such as buttons, pockets, and pipes. Machover states that the overall content and configuration of elements in drawings constitute what is most important; however, her work does not always support this premise. Although she insists that she did not intend to develop a list of singular elements linked to specific diagnoses, her material oftens appears to ascribe meanings authoritatively to certain characteristics. Machover did emphasize that the structural qualities (size, line, shading, and composition) in human figure drawings are more reliable than parts of the body, clothing, or other details, but overall her work in the area of person drawings has not been empirically validated and seems to be solely based on clinical observations.

Koppitz (1968), who constructed developmental scoring systems for children's drawings, seems to concur with Machover's ideas with regard to self-concept. She observes that a human figure a child draws, regardless of whom he or she draws, is a reflection of the child's inner representation of self:

> The nonspecific instruction to draw a whole person seems to lead the child to look into himself and into his own feelings when trying to capture the essence of a person. The person a child knows best is himself; his picture of a person becomes therefore a portrait of his inner self, of his attitudes. (p. 5)

Koppitz's research on drawing with children was generally considered a tool for assessment of intelligence, although she also was interested in the evauation of personality. Her analysis of children's figure drawings differs from other drawing tests in that she created separate scales to determine developmental level and emotional indicators. She assembled a list of "developmental items," visual aspects that appear relatively rarely in young children, but show up more frequently with age; many of the items included are based on the early work of Goodenough (1926). According to Koppitz, these items appear in the drawings of all children by around the age of 10 years.

Koppitz's initial studies were with children ages 5 to 12 years, establishing tables for specific characteristics for children at various age levels. She later expanded her studies to include the human figure drawings of children up to 14 years, observing that detail in human figure drawings does not systematically increase past age 11.

Koppitz also worked on the use of drawings as projective tasks with children, looking for traits in children's drawings that were indications of emotional problems. She describes 30 specific characteristics of drawings that might be denotative of emotional conflicts, focusing on such aspects as the quality of the drawing (symmetry, shading, and integration) and the presence of unusual traits or absence of expected traits at various ages. However, unlike Machover, Koppitz did not use traditional psychoanalytic theory as her framework. She instead used Sullivan's theory of interpersonal relationship, a philosophy that emphasized ego psychology as well as conscious processes. In contrast to Machover's views, Koppitz was more interested in children's perspective of themselves and significant others and their attitudes toward their problems and conflicts. This philosophy was more "present-centered" in that it examined children's current status and feelings along with developmental, interpersonal, and emotional factors.

Others have also attempted to define and refine the projective aspects of children's drawings and other art expressions. Although there are many such individuals, a couple of authors in particular are worth noting. Alschuler and Hattwick (1947) observed the connections between personality and how young children paint. They related preschoolers' experiences with a brush, paint, and paper on an easel to impulse control and interpersonal skills and to expression of concerns and feelings. Their work, although significant in that it underscored developmental aspects of children's painting and personality, was limited in scope and population and suffered in its methodology. DiLeo (1970, 1973, 1983) also considered children's drawings to be aids in diagnosis of psychological problems. The conclusions DiLeo offers are less specific than those of Machover, Buck, and Koppitz, but they are noteworthy in that DiLeo attempts to link children's drawings with theories of art, human development, and personality.

Problematic Aspects of Projective Drawing Tests

Projective uses of drawings, particularly the work of Machover and Koppitz, have come under fire by many researchers and clinicians who believe that drawings are not easily classified by characteristics and that projective drawing tests do not take into consideration the multi-dimensional aspects of children. Many take issue with projective drawing findings, noting the problematic aspects of clinical interpretation of children's drawings (Golomb, 1990; Martin, 1988; Roeback, 1968; Swenson, 1968). For example, the literal interpretation of signs as presented by authors such as Machover, Koppitz, and others reduces understanding drawings to matching details and omissions to often singular meanings. This one-to-one approach of associating graphic characteristics with meaning is at best very limited.

Although studies of both the emotional and cognitive aspects of drawings of children continue to be explored, there has been no definite consensus about the meaning and purpose of art expressions and no singular, reliable way to interpret content. There have also been questions and concern about trying to interpret or accurately describe something as complex as an art product, particularly from lists of individual characteristics, omitted features, or unusual artistic details. To a great extent, projective drawing tasks have also lacked emphasis or recognition of what aspects may indeed be normal traits in children's drawings. Golomb (1990) also notes that little attention is paid to developmental aspects of drawings that allow the therapist to understand which characteristics are normal and which may be significant or important. Although some therapists continue to interpret children's drawings from information derived from projective drawing tasks, it is a flawed approach because it does not take into consideration the multidimensionality of art expressions and the children who create them.

There also has been uneasiness about the predominantly psychoanalytic slant of most projective drawings tasks when is comes to evaluating children. Analyzing art expression from a psychoanalytic perspective may be reductionist and prescriptive, limiting possibilities of looking at children's work from other perspectives that might give a more complete, less biased view of the child. For example, Machover's assumptions, although often quoted and applied to work with children, have not held up well under scrutiny, and several studies have criticized the idea that human figure drawings strictly represent personality, particularly conflicts, anxieties, and other emotional difficulties in children and adults (Roeback, 1968; Swenson, 1968). This underscores the problematic issue in using projectives: In many cases, they are solely used to identify pathology, rather than to present a more broadly based view.

Issues of validity and reliability in projective drawing tasks have also been raised (Martin, 1988; Malchiodi, 1994). Most studies found in the literature have not undergone review or reestablishment of norms for many years, often decades. Another criticism that projective drawing tests have received is their lack of sensitivity to culture, gender, class, and other factors. For example, using drawing tasks to measure children's intelligence is probably more a measure of how well the child meets the standards of Western culture rather than general intelligence. There may be aspects of gender bias, in that thes drawing tasks are designed to assess intelligence, emphasize cognition, body awareness, and emotional expression from a limited perspective. Also, many studies of projective drawing tests have used adult samples, and some clinicians mistakenly apply this information to work with children.

The emergence and continued clinical application of projective drawing tests have raised the question of whether it is appropriate to use art expressions to diagnose children. This concern about interpretation of children's drawings to identify diagnosable pathology is not new, however; in her early studies of children's human figure drawings, Goodenough (1926) warned those who used her drawing test with children about the limitations of using art expression for diagnosis. She emphatically stated that "the facts herein reported by no means intended to convey the impression that the writer is able to diagnose psychopathic tendencies in children by means of drawing. No such claim is justified" (p. 24). Her observation that children's drawings cannot and perhaps should not be used to diagnose pathology emphasizes that art expressions are not easily categorized by singular characteristics and that therapists who use projective tasks must respect the individual meanings of children's expressive work.

MULTIDIMENSIONAL APPROACHES TO UNDERSTANDING CHILDREN'S DRAWINGS

It is obvious that projective drawing tests and psychoanalytically based philosophies have had a significant impact on how children's drawings are viewed by therapists during this century. However, there are many other theoretical viewpoints that have important implications in a more complete understanding of children's art expressions. Although the information obtained from some projective drawing tests can provide a limited view of children's personality, development, and cognitive abilities, a more comprehensive way of looking at children's art is obviously necessary to address the multidimensional aspects of their expressive work. Since most therapists use drawing with children in therapeutic settings rather than diagnostic ones, additional ways of understanding how children communicate through art expression are often both necessary and helpful.

Communication, Expression, and Problem Solving

Psychologists, therapists, counselors, and others have long used drawings in less formal ways with children, ways that are not specifically designed to assess, diagnose, or evaluate the child, but to provide a way for the child to communicate issues, feelings, and other experiences, and to explore, invent, and problem solve through self-expression. One figure who stands out in the search for alternative ways to think about children's art is Rudolph Arnheim (1969, 1972, 1974). Arnheim, a psychologist, took a different stance in his consideration of art expression, moving away from the idea that children's artwork was solely an index of intelligence or that drawings simply represented the emotional conflicts of the maker, a belief supported by the psychoanalytic influences predominant during the 1940s and 1950s. He became an important force in a more art-based view of children's artistic activity, seeing the importance of both aesthetics and cognition and the interplay between media and development of ideas through visual form. As Golomb (1990) notes:

> It is to the credit of Rudolph Arnheim that students of child art have been able to free themselves from the conceptual straitjacket that narrowed our vision of the nature of child art and how it can be studied.

His work has laid a foundation for a new psychology of the arts and provided the necessary conceptual tools for analyzing child art as a symbolic domain that has its own intrinsic rules and developmental coher-
ence. (p. 2)

Over the last several decades, there has been renewed interest in
looking at children's drawings not only for the purpose of assessment
and evaluation but also for their importance in therapy and treatment. Significant to this trend in defining how children's art expressions can enhance therapeutic intervention is the emergence of the
field of art therapy. During the early 20th century, interest in the
meaning of symbols and images in art in psychiatry, psychology, and
education stimulated the development of the field of art therapy in
the late 1940s and 1950s. Since that time, art therapists have been inquisitive about the meaning of artistic expressions and have had an
increasingly strong impact on interest in and understanding of children's artwork created in therapy. The focus of art therapy has not
only been on deciphering the meaning of children's expressive work,
but also in comprehending the complexities of both the process and
product in art making. Most importantly, in contrast to early applications of projective drawings that focus largely on the graphic characteristics of the image, art therapists, although interested in the image
itself, have also encouraged children to say something about their
drawings. This insistence on receiving input from the child who created the work implies that children's perspectives are important to the
therapist's understanding and that children's art expressions have personal meaning.

The introduction of art therapy as a profession in the United
States is attributed to Margaret Naumburg in the 1940s, although
there may have been several other individuals exploring similar ideas
during the same time period (Junge & Asawa, 1994). Naumburg made
many significant contributions to the understanding of children's art,
beginning with her early explorations of artistic expression in work
with children at Walden, a progressive school in New York City that
emphasized the importance of the unconscious in education. At
Walden, Naumburg encouraged children to learn through spontaneous art expression in contrast to the prevailing traditional approaches involving a standardized curriculum.

As a result of her interests in psychoanalysis and her experiences
teaching art to children at Walden, Naumburg came to see art as a

form of symbolic speech and conclude that spontaneous art expression was useful in psychotherapeutic treatment (Naumburg, 1947, 1966). In contrast to the work with projective drawings tests that began earlier in the century, Naumburg made some important distinctions about the meaning and value of art in her work with children and adults. First, she saw art expression in therapy as a form of symbolic communication between the client and the therapist. More importantly, she noted the value of spontaneously produced art rather than images that resulted from specifically designed tests, something that not only separated the field of art therapy apart from other fields, but also set the stage for broader applications and ways of understanding children's visual expressions.

Naumburg's views of art expression were consonant with the time in that she saw it as a way to manifest unconscious imagery, an observation consistent with the predominant psychoanalytic viewpoint of the early 20th century. In the same vein, she also believed that imagery of both children and adults expressed their inner conflicts in a visual form. Cane (1951), an art educator and the sister of Margaret Naumburg, also realized the connection between emotions and the creative act of art making. She developed methods to help children draw and paint spontaneously through the use of music, movement, sound, and scribbling. Her work with children supported not only the idea that art expression was a release of unconscious material, but also that specific methods combining art and other modalities were conducive to this release. The ideas that both Naumburg and Cane explored formed the basis for subsequent development of art therapy with children, particularly in work and understanding of children's spontaneous imagery.

A few years after Naumburg, Edith Kramer, an artist, educator, and pioneer in the field of art therapy, pointed to another important component inherent to art making with children. Kramer (1993) believed that the healing potentialities of art therapy reside in the psychological processes that are activated in creative work. She stressed creativity, not merely communication of visually symbolic speech, as key to use of the art process with children in therapy.

Kramer's philosophy developed in the 1930s, when she gave art classes in Prague for children of refugees of Nazi Germany (Junge & Asawa, 1994), learning the value and meaning of art expression with traumatized children. She later worked in school and residential treatment programs, realizing that children's art expression in therapy was a form of sublimation, an act of transforming impulses and emotions into images. One of Kramer's many contributions to therapeutic work with children's art expressions is her exploration of how the therapist can assist a child in self-expression through art by teaching developmentally appropriate art skills, serving as a responsive and reflective person in therapy, and even serving as a "third hand" in intervening and supporting the child's creative process of artistic expression. This philosophical contribution to understanding children's art expressions created in therapy deemphasizes the passive, silent stance of the psychoanalytic observer who does not interfere or intervene in the drawing process.

In Great Britain, pediatrician Donald Winnicott (1971) explored the idea that children's art could be used as a means of communication between therapist and child. He developed a technique similar to the scribble drawings of Naumburg and Cane that he called the "squiggle game" in which the child and therapist create a scribble (i.e., squiggle) through drawing together. Winnicott would draw a squiggle on paper that the child would then elaborate upon and transform into something else. The child would then draw a second squiggle that the therapist would then embellish to create an image. The technique's purpose was to initiate communication of the child's inner thoughts and feelings and could be used as a way for the child to tell a story about the images created. However, the squiggle game was not designed to be a projective drawing task per se; rather, it emphasized drawing as a catalyst for communication between therapist and child to help the child develop personal metaphors through art expression. An intuitive approach rather than one based in identifying specific features or details was used by Winnicott to explore and determine the content of the squiggle drawings, underscoring the child's important role in the communication of meaning.

Drawing, Play, and Development

Winnicott's technique is one of many developed in play therapy, a field that has peripherally added to the collective knowledge of children's drawings. Play has been used in child therapy since the 1920s (A. Freud, 1926, 1946) and employs games, toys, and art materials to build relationships with children, interpret children's behavior, assist children in trauma and distress, and support growth and change.

Many play therapists use drawing and other art activities in their work with children (Gil, 1991; Webb, 1991), often as an adjunct to other play activity. Sometimes this use of art activity is purposeful; that is, children are encouraged to draw a picture of their choice or are given a directive to make a specific image. Other therapists may use a more spontaneous way of working, allowing the child to move from play activity to art making and back again. Play therapists, psychologists, or counselors who use play in their work with children generally see children's drawings as nonverbal communication, as graphic representations of problems, and as an enhancement of the play therapy process. Although, except from anecdotal records, there have been few research data in the field of play therapy on how drawings can be specifically used to understand children, the collective work of play therapists who use art in their work emphasizes the important links between art and play and the significance of that connection on the process of children's artistic expression.

Drawings and art expressions of children have been examined from perspectives that began to include multidisciplinary approaches to understanding. Rubin (1984a, 1984b), an art therapist and psychologist, integrated art therapy, creative play, art education, and psychotherapy in her work with children. Her work with normal, emotionally disturbed, special needs, and handicapped children emphasizes a broad understanding of how children use art for many purposes—for mastery, for self-expression, for self-definition, and for addressing stress, emotional problems, and trauma through art. Rubin's philosophy about understanding children through their art underscores both the innate abilities of children to grow through artistic expression and how the therapist can facilitate this process.

Others have looked at children's art expressions from diverse perspectives and interests, integrating philosophies of artistic development, art education, art therapy, and psychotherapy, including: developmental considerations with relation to special needs and handicapping conditions (Anderson, 1992; Henley, 1992); the impact of trauma, particularly violence and abuse (Cohen & Phelps, 1985; Malchiodi, 1990, 1997); Jungian approaches and symbolic communication (Allan, 1988); and fixation on particular stages of artistic development (Levick, 1983, 1986).

Studies of the form and content of art expressions of young children from biological, human developmental, and anthropological sources have greatly added to the understanding of children's drawings from perspectives not solely psychologically based. Developmental perspectives are among the most widely examined, establishing the possibility of universal developmental stages in children's artistic expression. Viktor Lowenfeld (1947; Lowenfeld & Brittain, 1982), one of the most widely read art educators of this century, noted that children's intellectual growth was connected to creative development and delineated a well-known sequence of predictable stages of artistic development in children, a continuation of earlier work on the subject by Cooke (1885), Burt (1921), and others. In addition to artistic development, Lowenfeld (1947) also saw the value of art in self-expression:

> The process of drawing, painting or constructing is a complex one in which the child brings together diverse elements of his environment to make a meaningful whole. In the process of selecting, interpreting and reforming these elements, he has given us more than a picture, he has given us a part of himself. (p. 1)

Some (e.g., Gardner, 1980, and Winner, 1982) have continued Lowenfeld's and other's work in the area of art making and child development. Winner (1982) emphasizes that children's art expressions are quite complex, even at very young ages and that the development of drawing is not a simple, straightforward matter. Both Gardner and Winner stress the relationship of children's drawings to the development of cognitive abilities.

Integrating the fields of child development and anthropology, Kellogg (1969) observed the occurrence of specific patterns common to all human beings, universal images that are expressed by children through similar formal structures. Her collection and study of over 200,000 children's drawings demonstrated the common forms, shapes, and configurations that appear in young children's art. Kellogg's comprehensive study traced children's pictorial development from their first attempts to make marks on paper to when they begin to draw representational objects such as humans, animals, trees, and houses. Others have introduced the idea that there is a biological reason for art making, and, to some extent, this connection has an impact on the drawing activities of children (Morris, 1962; Dissanayake, 1989).

Silver (1978, 1988, 1996a) has devoted over 20 years to understanding the role of art in intellectual and emotional development. In her early work with deaf children and later with the learning disabled and adult stroke victims, she takes a cognitive approach to analyzing children's drawings, observing that cognitive skills can be assessed and developed through certain art tasks. According to Silver, children's drawings are images that can reflect their thinking vicariously as well as economically in the sense that a few lines and forms can represent an idea, figure, environment, or concept. The Silver Drawing Test and subsequent research by Silver demonstrate that drawing can indicate the ability to sequence, to represent spatial relationships of height, width, and depth, and the ability to select and combine in a creative way. Her work supports the idea that art expression can provide important information on these three areas of cognitive development, areas not previously addressed in early projective and other drawing tests. More recently, Silver has used stimulus drawings to investigate childhood depression and gender differences (1996a).

The impact of the growth of art therapy and therapists' inclusion of art therapy techniques in their work with children have underscored the importance of drawings as communications from child to therapist. The trend in the field of art therapy has been to emphasize the importance of the person who created the drawing to define, explore, and ultimately to assist the therapist in determining its meaning. This way of looking at art expressions has deemphasized the view that drawings are simply conglomerations of characteristics to be dissected or connected to singular meanings. Instead, this philosophy is more consonant with the practical day-to-day practice of child therapists who work with children and their art not only to understand the meaning of children's images, but also to provide art activity as therapeutic intervention for the child.

Also, in contrast to projective drawing tasks, the field of art therapy has spent more energy on looking at the spontaneous drawings and art expressions of children, in addition to drawings that are responses to specific drawing tasks or tests. These efforts, although they have yielded little quantifiable data, have generated a more comprehensive view and respect for the multifacted aspects of art expressions. They have emphasized that looking at drawings is not a cut and dry matter, but one which requires a broader view of art making. An understanding not only of psychological aspects is necessary as well as aspects of the art process, materials, and changes in children's art expressions over time.

Currently, researchers in the field of art therapy are exploring ways to understand drawings through the structural qualities of art expression, the art-making process, and the effects of materials, rather than specific items, elements, or omissions as in projective drawing tasks. For example, Gantt and Tabone (1998) have developed an assessment tool that takes into consideration the structure of art expression, rather than focusing on the individual characteristics themselves. Likewise, Cohen and Cox (1995) have also developed an integrative approach to understanding art expressions through structural characteristics, process, and content. Although these ways of looking at the qualities of art expression have focused on the art expressions of adults, both approaches hold promise for new ways of looking at children's drawings and other creative work and could impact the ways in which children's drawings are understood.

CONCLUSION

This short chapter has provided a brief overview of the diverse philosophies that clinicians and researchers have developed to try to decipher, define, and understand children's drawings. Historically, the majority of what has been written for helping professionals on children's art has focused largely on projective drawing tasks or tests, reflecting the early connections between psychoanalytic thought and the symbolic meanings of images. Although some of this information may support certain general trends in children's drawings, most of this evidence shows that tests are limited in scope on their own and that there are only weak connections between single graphic characteristics and personality and affect. Overall, this material has focused on aspects of personality with an emphasis on problems and pathology and, in an effort to quantify drawings, has sacrificed a great deal of the complexities of children's art.

What is important to remember is that there are many dimensions and many possible theoretical frameworks to consider. Most of all, it is essential to respect children's visual communications for all their richness, uniqueness, complexity, and spontaneity. Children's art expressions, like children themselves, are individual and must be considered as such and within the larger context of their developmental, emotional, social, and cultural experiences.

While projective drawings and other art-based assessments have been used for evaluation purposes, most helping professionals are looking to art expressions not only for information in order to be best able to intervene or plan therapeutic intervention, but also as interventions in and of themselves. In reality, most therapists will be using children's drawings in other ways than for assessment purposes, adding art activities to therapy as a way for children to problem solve, to express feelings and perceptions, and to work through situations, memories, or emotions that are troubling them. Art expression, in this sense, is not really a means of diagnostic evaluation per se, but a modality for allowing children to relate their experiences in an age-appropriate manner. When drawing is used as a part of therapy, it is not necessary or possible to apply information from drawings tasks designed as for evaluation or diagnosis, since the goal is therapeutic intervention rather than assessment.

Lastly, most therapists and clinicians will likely be looking at children's drawings in addition to other material, such as behavioral observations, psychological assessments, and self-reports. Art expression may supplement or support this information, or may, in most cases, serve a way for the child to communicate and participate in therapy through a creative task. Projective drawing tasks arguably have had some problems and pitfalls in terms of reliability of research. However, alternative ways of understanding art expressions, as presented in this chapter, have been based largely on clinical observations and, to date, have not been carefully researched. Despite inherent problems in our understanding, defining, and comprehending children's creative work, the continuing interest in children's drawings as reflections of their inner worlds underscores therapists' ongoing fascination with children's art expressions and the consensus that drawings are undeniably important in both evaluation and therapeutic work with children.

CHAPTER TWO

Children's Drawings in Context

For children, art making is a process that brings together many different experiences to create something new, personal, and unique. The process of making a drawing requires the child to choose, translate, and arrange lines, shapes, and colors to convey a thought, feeling, event, or observation, synthesizing numerous components involving content, style, form, and composition. Because so many different elements and experiences come together in children's drawings, simple explanations and interpretations of their creative work are not always possible.

For those helping professionals who have not had much personal experience with art, looking at children's drawings may be seen as a mystifying task or unfortunately, as a simple process that involves checking for specific characteristics that indicate problems or pathology. In actuality, viewing drawings as mystifying is probably more helpful to children in the long run, since at least one is looking at children's work with an open mind. Seeing children's art expressions simply as a series of components and diagnostic characteristics is much more problematic and does not take into consideration the context in which they were created or the possibility of multi-meaning. In using this limited approach, therapists may look at art expressions only with intent to analyze them, make assumptions, categorize them, or sometimes even pathologize them. As Rubin (1984b) notes, "Even if it turns out that one's initial guess about meaning was correct, one should not assume that any image 'always' means something specific, nor even that its significance is invariant over time for any particular person" (p. 128).

As an art therapist who has looked at children's drawings for over

20 years, I am somewhat conservative about making specific determinations or speculations concerning the content of a child's drawing or art expressions. The experience of childhood is in some ways universal, but is also quite variable when one considers the many environmental influences such as culture, class, gender expectations, and parenting, and the genetic determinants that affect children. For children the process of art making is also shaped by a variety of factors in addition to biopsychosocial factors. These include the materials with which children draw, the environment in which they create, and their personal capacities, motivations, talents, or interests in drawing or art making. The child's relationship with the helping professional will also affect the content and style of drawing, including the level of trust and safety between child and adult and the therapist's sensitivity to the process of drawing and understanding of artistic activity in children.

Also introduced in this chapter is the importance of taking a phenomenological view of children's drawings. In order to avoid imposing adult standards on children's work and making assumptions about content and meaning, I believe that the therapist has to be open to a variety of meanings in drawings as well as to the child's unique way of viewing the world. This final section addresses the need to consider children's art from many perspectives in order to develop a more integral view of children's drawings made in therapy.

WHAT MOTIVATES CHILDREN TO DRAW?

In order to understand children's approaches to drawing or other creative expression, it is first important to consider what motivates their spontaneous expressions. There are usually three ways that children arrive at the images they draw: memory, imagination, and life.

Memory, Imagination, and Real Life

Drawings from memory are based on what children recall about the object, person, animal, or environment that they are asked to draw or choose to try to recall through drawing. Drawing from memory is not particularly easy for all children (or adults, for that matter). For example, when asked to draw a family, a popular request by many therapists who work with children, many children will make very simple figures without much detail. Sometimes in order to obtain more detailed drawings of themes such as families, a bit of coaching and encouragement is needed to get any kind of a response on paper at all.

Therapists often ask children to draw something from their imagination, such as images of feelings or make-believe stories. For some children, this will come easily, and they will be able to create drawings that have original and interesting themes, whereas others may be somewhat lost and not able to put on paper anything imaginative or novel. This can be particularly true for children who have been chronically abused or traumatized to the point of psychological numbness; it is often difficult for these children to call forth anything to put on paper. Other children may just fear failure in trying to create something without any guidelines or assistance. There is also concern that children's preoccupation with television and video games has decreased their abilities to be imaginative through art expression (Kramer, Gerity, Henley, & Williams, 1995), although no quantifiable evidence for this supposition has been gathered.

It is important to acknowledge that many children simply find it difficult to come up with something strictly from their imagination. Gardner (1982) notes that some young children require little stimulation to begin artistic work (self-starters), whereas others, when presented with art materials and an attentive adult, were more reluctant to begin work. The latter group may feel more uncertain about how to proceed, anxious, or self-conscious about the situation or adult watching them. However, if given a product to complete (such as an unfinished drawing or design), they can often create a work even more inventive than the self-starters.

Developmental factors can affect children's inclination to be imaginative. For example, older children and adolescents may prefer to copy something or look at something around them, since developmentally this is a time that children feel strongly about making a picture look real and often are concerned about having the correct details. Although they may be able to create a drawing from imagination, they can be uncomfortable with "making a mistake" or may be disappointed in the results of their drawings. Young children, in contrast, are generally more spontaneous and are less concerned with photographically accurate details in their drawings.

The third way children draw is by looking at objects in the real world—in other words, drawing something that is right in front of them. Although therapists may not ask children to draw something that they see in the immediate environment, children may choose to make a drawing of something they see in the world around them. As previously noted, older children and adolescents are more likely to be interested in this type of drawing because developmentally, they are concerned with getting details to be realistic, correct, and photographic.

Attitudes about Drawing

Attitudes about drawing and art making are often shaped in childhood, and what a therapist communicates to a child about his or her drawings can have a long-lasting impact. In my clinical work with adults who consider themselves to be nonartists, I often hear them recall a particular memory from childhood that formed their current perspective on art and their ability to be an artist. Art expression is a very personal creative endeavor, and both children and adults are vulnerable to disparaging remarks about their art. Even when the remarks are meant to be noncritical, but are perceived as negative or criticizing, an individual may find them intimidating or inhibiting. Many adults recall with vivid detail the time that the classroom teacher displayed art that was judged to be good out in the hall for others to admire and their art on the back of the door to the classroom, meaning it was not good. Remarks made by parents can have an impact on children's desire and motivation to make art; even the most well-meaning parent has, on occasion, misinterpreted the content of a child's drawing, perhaps unknowingly discouraging the child from continuing to draw. These statements and actions can and do affect the content, style, and quality of visual expression, and certainly children's capacity and interest in art making.

Experiences with Art Making

Many people do not believe that previous experiences with art activities have a significant effect on children's drawings and their content. However, there are several experiences that seem to have at least some effect on what and how children draw. One powerful influence on the content and style of artwork is how children are taught art.

Some children may become dependent on props such as coloring books and predrawn images provided by well-meaning adults or classroom teachers. For example, children who are given coloring books or predrawn images may adopt these images in lieu of inventing their own unique drawings. Figure 2.1 shows a drawing of a bird by a 4-year-old girl before exposure to coloring books. Figure 2.2 is the book illustration that the child was given to color in school, and Figure 2.3 is

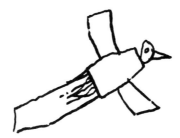

FIGURE 2.1. Drawing of a bird by a 4-year-old girl before exposure to coloring book. From *Artforms* by Diane and Sarah Preble. Copyright 1985 by Addison-Wesley Educational Publishers, Inc. Reprinted by permission.

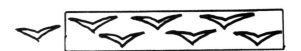

FIGURE 2.2. Illustrations of birds in a coloring book. From *Artforms* by Diane and Sarah Preble. Copyright 1985 by Addison-Wesley Educational Publishers, Inc. Reprinted by permission.

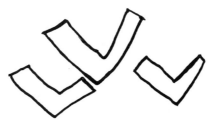

FIGURE 2.3. A girl's drawing of birds after exposure to coloring book birds. From *Artforms* by Diane and Sarah Preble. Copyright 1985 by Addison-Wesley Educational Publishers, Inc. Reprinted by permission.

her drawing of birds after exposure to the coloring book. Children do repeat these stereotypic images in their own visual work, finding it difficult to come up with ideas of their own or develop an individual mode of expression. Others may become fixed on a particular way or strategy for drawing that was taught to them. It is common to see at least some stereotypic images in children's art expressions because most children are taught something about drawing or given coloring tasks in school that have a long-lasting influence on how and what they draw in other situations.

Some children may be influenced through art shown to them by adults. An exhibit of hospitalized children's art at a hospital in the community where I live featured an image a child had painted that was described as illustrating abuse the child had experienced from violent parents. The image created by the child was powerful and dramatic: a picture of a wounded deer with a human head. The child had, in fact, copied a famous painting by the Mexican artist Frida Kahlo, one that includes the body of a deer impaled with arrows and the head of the artist. Although the choice of the child to copy this image may have been significant, the art instructor's own interest in the painting and use of this image in the art program had a probable impact on the child's choice to copy it. Despite the provocative content of the child's drawing, the influence of the art teacher and the art shown the child as inspiration had guided the work rather than it being a spontaneous expression by the child.

Sociocultural Influences

Lastly, sociocultural influences can affect children's motivation to draw and their attitudes about art making in general. Culture can also influence the content of children's art expressions, although there has been relatively little research exploring cultural aspects of drawings (Alland, 1983; Dennis, 1966). How race, ethnicity, socioeconomic status, and religion affect children's motivations and attitudes about drawing has not been explored extensively, but nevertheless, these are likely to be an important influence on their creative work.

In my travels to other countries, the differences in how children respond to requests to draw have been the most dramatic. Many years ago I was invited to China to train therapists to use art as therapy with children and adults. As part of my assignment I worked with several groups of 6- and 7-year-old children in schools around Beijing. Although their artwork was developmentally comparable to children's drawings in the United States, the children were not comfortable with being asked to draw spontaneously, preferring that I draw a picture for them to copy. This was not surprising because their beliefs about art activity involved receiving instruction on how to draw by the adult in authority rather than developing ideas of their own. In contrast to most American children I had worked with, the Chinese children I interacted with were extremely quiet, attentive, and more reserved, characteristics that a therapist in the United States might perceive as being shy or even withdrawn. However, through their silence and deference, this particular group of Chinese children were showing me respect, an important quality within their culture.

Other sociocultural influences may come from what a child learns at home about art activities and about interacting with adults in general. A child who appears reserved when asked to draw may have been taught at home to respect the adult in authority, to be careful not to make a mess or to waste materials, or to wait for instructions and approval before proceeding. Differences in race or cultural background between therapist and child may also be a factor in a child's willingness to comply with requests to draw, just as ethnocultural differences have been highlighted as important to therapeutic interventions in general (Campanelli, 1991; Pinderhughes, 1989). These differences as well as learned beliefs and values are important to decipher and understand before developing any conclusions about a child's interest, motivation, and process of drawing.

DRAWING AS A PROCESS

Very few therapists who use drawing with children, with the exception of art therapists, probably have ever given any conscious thought to what drawing is and its unique characteristics as an art process. However, it is important to understand what you are assigning children to do when asking them to draw and what children perceive drawing to be from their developmental point of view. Because it is vital for the therapist to fully understand what the process of drawing entails, the following section is included for therapists unfamiliar with art processes and drawing materials. Of course, the best way to understand drawing is to experience it first hand. Reading about drawing is like watching people swim and expecting to know what the experience is like by only observing it; you have to get into the water to fully understand the experience.

Drawing, in its simplest sense, is the depiction of forms, shapes, and images with lines. It often involves using a drawing instrument of some kind to make marks on paper, although one can draw lines in the sand or even through the air with one's fingers. Drawing for children involves both a process (making of art) and a product (the completed art expression). It is on the latter, the product, that helping professionals who seek to understand more about their child clients, often place most of their focus. However, in order truly to begin to understand the meaning of drawing for children, the process of drawing must also be thoroughly understood.

Kramer (1971) provides a comprehensive description of the various ways that children use art materials in the process of drawing, painting, and creating. According to her observations, there are five ways in which art materials may be used:

1. Precursory activities: scribbling, smearing, exploration of physical properties of the material that does not lead to creation of symbolic configurations but is experienced as positive and egosyntonic.
2. Chaotic discharge: spilling, splashing, pounding, destructive behavior leading to loss of control.
3. Art in the service of defense: stereotyped repetition; copying, tracing, banal conventional production.
4. Pictographs: pictorial communications which replace or supplement words.
5. Formed expression, or art in the full sense of the word: the production of symbolic configurations that successfully serve both self-expression and communication. (pp. 54–55)

Kramer's description is important because it not only enhances understanding of the art product but also the art process in work with children and their drawings. For example, many children, for various reasons, will engage in drawing activities that do not lead to actual finished art expressions. Sometimes this is simply, as Kramer (1971) describes, experimentation with materials; for example, when learning about what clay can do, a child may pound, twist, roll, or draw lines in the clay in order to explore its possibilities. Some children may be unproductive for other reasons. Anxious, nervous, hyperactive, or emotionally overwhelmed children may quickly engage in chaotic discharge, particularly if the task is not structured and materials are not carefully chosen. For example, a hyperactive 10-year-old child may end up scribbling unproductively or a traumatized 7-year-old may crumple or tear paper rather than experiment with materials and work on a well-formed image because of an inability to become focused on drawing.

In other situations, the combination of children's personalities, materials, and tolerance for the activity presented can create similar results. For example, a graduate student I was supervising wanted to engage a group of children in a large painting project with tempera paints on mural paper. His idea focused on a story he would read to the children about calling each other on the telephone; the children would then work together to paint telephone lines to each other on the paper, simulating calling each other by phone. I immediately sensed this might get out of hand, knowing that these children had just arrived at the facility and seemed agitated. I advised him about the possible problems of assigning this exercise to these children, but he was excited to try it anyway. Minutes after the activity began there was paint (and chaos) everywhere; the graduate student was obviously depressed with the results. The reaction of the children was mixed; some were frustrated and annoyed, whereas others found great pleasure in regressing with paint. What resulted was a miserable mess of paint on paper rather than any well-formed expression or content.

It is easy to see that the watery, uncontrollable paint utilized in an activity involving movement can provide an environment for chaos to develop rapidly. In this example, the children were already in a state of substantial excitement, and the activity raised that to the level of pandemonium. Paint, by its very nature, can elicit affective material, and in combination with a rather kinesthetic activity (the making of lines across a large paper), it can become very regressive. In some situations, these qualities may be desirable; for example, a child who is very reserved or feels an excessive need for control and structure may benefit from the experience of playing with materials in a supportive environment.

THE IMPORTANCE OF MATERIALS

In order for drawing to take place, both materials and a place to draw are necessary. These may seem like two obvious components to the process of drawing, but some therapists who use art activities with children may not have considered the importance of materials used to draw and the environment or space in which drawing takes place. Both have a significant influence on the outcome of children's art expressions as well as their overall interest in drawing.

First, providing good quality materials with which to draw can affect the richness of the expressive material in children's drawings in terms of amount, quantity, and variety. For example, the condition of materials can influence how children choose and use color in a drawing. Some children will not under any circumstances use a crayon that is broken, preferring to use only those that are good condition and intact. In work with chalks or pastels, some children may only use those pastels that have a paper wrapper around them so that their fingers will not become soiled. Although this says something about the individual child's personality and preferences, it can affect how children select colors with which to draw and the content of their drawings.

It is equally important for the therapist to have a working knowledge of drawing materials. If a therapist is not familiar with art materials and what they can do, the child cannot be adequately instructed in how to use materials to make well-formed and expressive drawings. Personal experience with the art process cannot be overemphasized, and direct involvement with art materials is highly recommended as a way to truly understand materials because verbal observation will not adequately convey this information.

There are several qualities of materials that influence the content and style of children's drawings (for a more complete description of drawing materials, see the Appendix). The size of drawing paper, for example, is an important factor in how and what children draw. Standard white 8½″ × 11″ paper is often less threatening to children who are ovewhelmed by crisis (i.e., less space to fill) and may encourage more detailed drawings but also can be confining for others. Larger paper may encourage more movement and playful expression; however, because it can promote movement, it may be counterproductive to use with children who are manic or hyperactive in their behavior (as described in the previous example of the graduate student and the large painting project).

The color of the drawing paper also can affect the choice of color(s) children chose to draw with. Although most therapists generally think of white paper for drawing activities with children, it may be important to use a colored paper in some situations. For example, black paper is reported to be helpful to children with learning disabilities, perceptual problems, or visual impairments. The dark background provides a high contrast, expecially if the child is provided with a white crayon or chalk for drawing. This reversal of the usual object-ground materials (e.g., pencil or crayon on a white background) has been connected to enhancing children's abilities to articulate form and detail more easily (Uhlin, 1979).

It is important to say a few words about color and drawing materials at this point. First, the type of materials that children use to make drawings will directly affect the color in their drawings. Felt markers that provide bright and often bold colors will leave a more powerful impression than colored pencils, which tend to be rather light in value and difficult to color large areas. Some materials are also more easily blended than others; chalk or oil pastels are two media that can be blended, although many children will simply use pure color unless someone suggests to them to mix the colors together or has taught them this skill.

Rubin (1984a) nicely summarizes the importance of knowing, incorporating, and respecting materials in therapeutic work with children:

> If art materials are cared for lovingly by adults, they will not only remain most usable, but children will learn respect for the tools of the trade. . . . They must be appropriate for the children who are expected to use them—appropriate to their developmental level, degree of coordination, previous experiences, particular interests, and special needs. . . . If materials are of sufficient variety, then children may discover and develop their own unique tastes and preferences, their own favorite forms of expression. (pp. 30–31)

THE INFLUENCE OF ENVIRONMENT

Environment is another aspect that can have an impact on the content and style of children's drawings. When I was an elementary school art teacher, the two schools at which I worked provided some very different environments for art activities. At one school, I brought art activities to large classrooms of students with neat and orderly rows of chairs. In the other school, I met much smaller groups of children in a large meeting hall at tables. Although there were other factors that differentiated the students in these two schools, the space in which they created art certainly had an effect on their creative process. For the children in the crowded but orderly classroom, the art expressions were just as colorful and imaginative as other children's, but often the children in this environment were obsessively neat, carefully structuring and coloring their drawings. The school's philosophy was one of order and discipline, a philosophy that had an effect on the children. However, the constrictions of the space itself (in this case, a very structured classroom with limited movement) had a very recognizable impact on the style of the art.

The children at the other school had the freedom to move about and a great deal of space in which to move. Because of their less-restricted environment, they often engaged in spontaneous movement or singing while working on their art projects (at least as much as I could tolerate and still keep some order to the class). The children would often request to make large drawings or paintings and loved to act out their images for the group; in contrast, the children at the crowded, more orderly school preferred to share their art within a structured routine at the end of each class, involving one of the children holding up each drawing for group applause.

Although a space designed for drawing and other art activities is ideal, therapists often have to work with children in environments that serve other functions. In my work with traumatized children, I have held therapy sessions in a variety of spaces, depending on what was available: kitchens, TV lounges, recreation rooms (where the ping-pong table doubles as an art table), and occasionally, a real art room. At other times, I have had to use an office that was usually employed by social workers to interview clients. An adult desk or table is a common place for therapy in shelters and safe houses, but it is not particularly conducive for children's art activities. Adult furniture can be a deterrent to art making with children because it sets up an uncomfortable and difficult situation for drawing or other art activities.

Additionally, the child (and the therapist) constantly have the added worry of making a mess with chalks, paints, glue, or other art materials. If one of the interventional goals for the child is to help him or her to freely express through drawing, then this type of environment is not helpful in achieving such purposes. In order to get a child deeply involved in the process, at minimum, a table and chairs comfortable and suitable for children are important to their participation and ease of expression.

Space is undoubtedly a factor in children's expressiveness, and, as in the example described above, it is important to recognize how the immediate environment influences children's participation level and their images. Most therapists are aware that many children can be stimulated by a well-designed space but that others can be overwhelmed by too much space and distractions in the environment. Some children are easily excited by excessive amounts of materials and toys in the immediate vicinity, especially when they are anxious or upset to begin with, and this can reduce their ability to remain focused on drawing. Although in many circumstances therapists will not have complete control over the environment in which children draw, it is important to be cognizant of the influence of space on children's attentiveness and involvement in drawing experiences.

The environment in which art making takes place must also feel safe for the children to freely draw images that they may not want others to see. The circumstances for drawing should be as comfortable and as safe as possible in order to allow children the security they need. Many children who come to therapy are distressed, apprehensive, or fearful, and for these children, any new or unfamiliar environment is anxiety producing. In order to provide a safe place for art expression, it is necessary to have options for space to be alone with the therapist or far from others in a group or family situation. Since the very nature of therapy is confidential, the space used for drawing generally should be as private as it would be for any other therapeutic session. Because safety and confidentiality are prominent ethical issues in work with children, they will be discussed in more depth in Chapter 8.

CHILDREN'S DRAWING AND THE THERAPEUTIC RELATIONSHIP

One additional aspect of working with children and their drawings that is often overlooked is the effect of the relationship between the therapist and child on the child's art expression. This context—the interactions between a helping adult and a child who has the role of client in the relationship—is an important and powerful dynamic that can have an impact on the child's creative process. The child's relationship to the therapist and the stage of their relationship has a significant effect on what the child draws or feels free to express.

Most mental health professionals who work with children know that what works to make a healthy and productive relationship between adults will not necessarily work with children. Children's abilities to grasp concepts are less advanced than those of adults and therapists have to be careful to present interventions and activities in ways that are appropriate to their developmental level. For therapists who are trained in adult counseling skills, it is necessary to modify their approach and language when it comes to working with children. Moustakas (1959) describes the components of an effective relationship between therapists and children:

> a place where the normal child is able to release tensions and frustrations that accumulate in the course of daily living, to have materials and an adult entirely to himself, without any concern with sharing, being cooperative, being considerate, polite or mannerly. He can feel his feelings and express his thoughts all the way knowing that he is accepted and revered unconditionally. (p. 42)

Children, depending on their experiences and cultural background, may see the therapist as an authority figure, rule maker, or advisor, rather than a person who helps them to openly share their thoughts and feelings. Therapists who assign activities or ask questions in ways that are not congruent with children's development or who are overly intrusive may also seem imposing to children. They may be fearful or anxious in the presence of the therapist no matter how warm, caring, and sensitive the therapist may be. Children, as Moustakas notes, need to feel free to express themselves unreservedly, without fears, constraints, or defenses. Unconditional acceptance of images and establishment of free expression are also important to the process of art making in therapy.

Because developing a therapeutic relationship with children often takes time, it is unwise to jump to conclusions or meanings about the content of children's drawings until one examines one's impact on the child through the therapeutic dynamic. For example, many therapists assume that if a child draws a very small human figure at an initial evaluation or intake, the child may feel inadequate or withdrawn, or have a low sense of self-esteem; much of the literature on projective drawings supports this possibility. Sometimes a child will draw a figure as small as possible so the observing adult cannot see it or because the child is intimidated by the therapist or by the new situation. This reaction may be indicative of the way the child responds to other un-comfortable situations or people, but the reaction may also be a func-tion of the immediate relationship between therapist and child.

Children's drawings can also reflect the developing relationship between the therapist and child over the course of therapy. Figures 2.4, 2.5, and 2.6 provide interesting examples of what changes can take place in a child's expressions and how those expressions may re-flect changes in the relationship between child and therapist over even a very limited span of time. The drawings were done by a 5-year-old girl during an initial evaluation conducted by an art therapist at the safe house for battered women at which the girl was staying with her mother. She was asked three times during the hour to draw a house, tree and person; her first response was the crayon drawing in Figure 2.4 in which she very nervously and silently drew a tiny house (which she said had no doors), a small tree, and a person of similar size who is crying. As many children who come with their mothers to seek refuge from violence in the home, she was extremely fearful of this new and confusing situation and of the art therapist, a strange adult.

These feelings, however, would change over the course of the hour as she became less threatened and more comfortable with the therapist. Her second rendition (Figure 2.5) shows greater usage of the space, a larger house, and a smiling person. She spontaneously asked if a tree could be a flower instead, displaying increased comfort with the session and self-initiating an imaginative solution to the directive. In her third and final version (Figure 2.6), accomplished near the end of

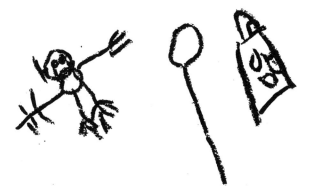

FIGURE 2.4. Initial drawing of a house, tree, and person by a 5-year-old girl. From *Breaking the Silence* by Cathy A. Malchiodi. Copyright 1997 by Brunner/Mazel. Reprinted by permission.

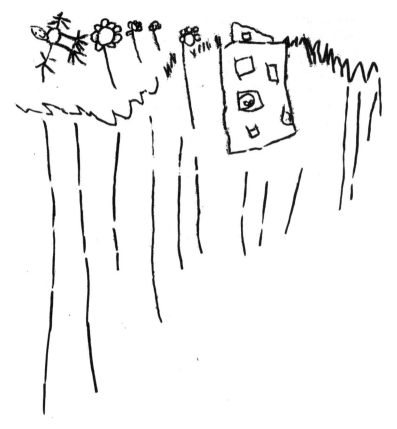

FIGURE 2.5. Second drawing of a house, tree, and person by a 5-year-old girl. From *Breaking the Silence* by Cathy A. Malchiodi. Copyright 1997 by Brunner/Mazel. Reprinted by permission.

the hour, the girl showed ease and openness in drawing. She also became more talkative and, when asked about her drawing, eagerly volunteered that the "sun was out and it's warm and there are lots of flowers." There is also a larger, smiling person in the upper lefthand corner of the paper. From these examples, it is easy to see that there can be a variety of responses in expression over a short time span that give an increasingly more complete picture of the child. These drawings also underscore the importance of obtaining a series of art expressions rather than relying on one drawing from which to make judgments.

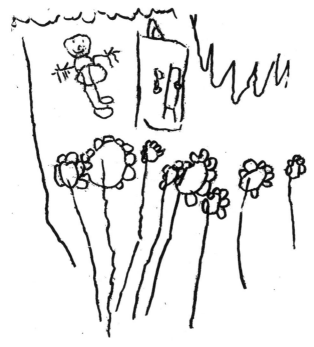

FIGURE 2.6. Third drawing of a house, tree, and person by a 5-year-old girl. From *Breaking the Silence* by Cathy A. Malchiodi. Copyright 1997 by Brunner/Mazel. Reprinted by permission.

A PHENOMENOLOGICAL APPROACH
TO UNDERSTANDING CHILDREN'S DRAWINGS

In order to address the contextual aspects previously mentioned and to avoid imposing adult standards on children's work and making assumptions about content and meaning, I prefer to use a phenomenological approach to understanding children and their drawings. Phenomenology is the study of events in their own right rather than from preconceived causes. What is important about a phenomenological approach to looking at children's drawings is its emphasis on an openness to a variety of meanings, the context in which they were created, and the maker's way of viewing the world. It is a way of understanding children's expressive work from many perspectives, allowing the viewer to amplify the images and construct meanings from more than one vantage point and to develop a more integral view of children's art expressions.

In its own right, phenomenology is a field of philosophy; however, it has become increasingly popular with researchers who want to approach data (in this case, children's drawings) without preconceived notions, expectations, or frameworks (Field & Morse, 1985). In the field of art therapy, it has been articulated best by Betensky (1995) in her work with clients and their art expressions:

> The centrality of the artmaker is one of the most essential factors. . . . The clients in art therapy, whose first-hand experience goes into the artmaking, are the chief beholders of their own art expressions. They are the ones who then experience the process of looking at the self-made phenomenon as it appears to their senses and consciousness. Thus, the artmakers themselves arrive at subjective meanings, not the art therapist. (p. 21)

Betensky diverts from true phenomenological observation, which includes only structural description of what one sees, and asks her clients to free associate with the content of their images and to come up with possible meanings. However, her approach underscores the importance of a client-centered, or in reference to work with children, a child-centered approach to understanding children's drawings respecting the child's responses in finding meaning in images. She also stresses humanistic aspects of art making as well as the gestalt qualities of art expression, saying, "While trait theory of personality assigns the individual into a diagnostic category and predicts his future behavior, and the psychodynamic personality model leans on the unconscious, both theories neglect the rich and illuminating variety of states of the conscious" (1995, p. 29).

In my own work with children's drawings from a phenomenological approach, the first step involves taking a stance of "not knowing." This is similar to the philosophy described by social constructivist theorists who see the therapist's role in work with people as one of cocreator, rather than expert advisor. By seeing the client as the expert on his or her own experiences, an openness to new information and discoveries naturally evolves for the therapist. Although art expressions may share some commonalities in form, content, and style, taking a stance of not knowing allows the child's experiences of creating and making art expressions to be respected as individual and to have a variety of meanings. In circumstances where therapists use cookbook approaches to catagorize images or a list of predetermined meanings for content, it is more likely that children's multiple or individual meanings will not be conveyed, will be misunderstood, and will possibly be disrespected.

A second feature of a phenomenological approach is the opportunity to acknowledge many different aspects of growth that are linked to art expression, including cognitive abilities, emotional development, interpersonal skills, and developmental maturity, and in my experience, somatic (physical) and spiritual aspects, subjects that will be addressed in subsequent chapters of this book. Children use art to integrate not only their inner experiences and perceptions, but also to link their experience of the outside world with the inner self, helping them to discover and affirm themselves and their relationships to people, environment, and even society. This multiplicity of meaning provides the therapist with material for developing and deepening the therapeutic relationship while also honoring the unique experiences of the child client from many perspectives. Although it may be difficult to truly understand all levels of meaning in children's expressive work, it is important to allow for the possibility of "multimeaning." As Rubin (1984b) notes, art has a potential to symbolize not only internal events, but interpersonal ones as well, and to condense many experiences, feelings, and perceptions into a single visual statement.

A phenomenological approach allows the therapist to comprehend children's drawings from an integral orientation rather than from a limited perspective. Many therapists unfortunately learn to rely on one or two theories in their thinking about clients. In my own training as an art therapist, I was originally taught to look at children's art expressions from developmental and emotional (mostly psychoanalytic) aspects. Since that time, experience with children has taught me that other aspects in addition to development and affect can be present in children's art, and if recognized and accepted, provide a more complete representation of the child's world.

One clinical example continues to be important in guiding my clinical work today and demonstrates that looking at children's work from narrow perspectives can limit the amount learned from children's drawings. In working with a little girl at a domestic violence shelter as her primary therapist, I was naturally concerned she may have experienced abuse from her father who had been reported to be violent to her mother and younger brother. Her drawings made during art therapy sessions at the facility particularly concerned me; each of them always contained a black center, particularly images of her body or human figures. This repetition of dark shading in her drawings led me to think that emotional or physical trauma might be rooted in this use of color. Since my training as an art therapist emphasized the emotional meanings of art expression, I naturally looked in that direction. However, this thinking obstructed other possible reasons as to why the child continued to use this characteristic in her work.

I later was surprised to learn that the girl had not been abused, but was indeed emotionally traumatized. She was so deeply traumatized, however, that she internalized her stress, and this in turn had caused her to develop a very painful stomach ulcer. When we later talked again about her drawings, she admitted to me that the black spots she included in each drawing were images of her physical pain, but she did not want to share this with anyone because of the trouble it might cause her mother and brother. In retrospect, if I had asked her about physical complaints rather than focusing solely on the emotional aspects of her traumatic situation, I may have considered other meanings for this repetitive use of black in her artwork.

Drawings generally have been routinely interpreted and even distorted through the singular use of psychological perspective or theory. For example, if a child draws a fish with an X-ray view of the contents of its stomach, a psychoanalytic view might see it as fears of being eaten by another or subconscious desires to devour something or someone. A cognitive view might focus on the thought process that went into making the drawing, investigating or speculating about what the child has recently seen (e.g., a nature show on television) or heard (e.g., the story of Jonah being swallowed by a fish). Another perspective may concentrate on the idea of metaphor, seeing the image as symbolic story unfolding, perhaps even archetypal in nature and representative of a universal theme or existential dilemma. In actuality, all of these approaches may contribute something important to one's overall understanding. Despite the problems inherent to projective drawing tasks and other systems of finding meaning in children's drawings, as Wilber (1996) notes about research in general, no one theory of understanding is completely wrong and "nobody is smart enough to be wrong all the time" (p. 13). In the case of children's art expressions, no one theory of interpreting or deciphering them is completely erroneous, and each does contribute some useful knowledge to understanding children's work.

Although a phenomenological approach is advantageous to understanding children's drawings, one cannot completely discount some of the more reliable information available relating specific content in children's drawings to certain meanings, experiences, and difficulties. This information can be useful, especially if used respectfully and as an additional perspective on children's art expressions. Many children, for various reasons, cannot or will not want to talk about their drawings. Some children will not talk simply because they cannot articulate their experiences with words. Others, particularly children seen in therapy, may feel threatened or afraid to tell their experiences, fearful of revealing a personal or family secret. Some may be concerned about what the therapist will think or do if they convey problems they are experiencing. For example, a 12-year-old girl I saw in my practice felt that she would be burdening the therapist with her problems because she saw the problems of her younger siblings as more important. Her assumption of the role of "caretaker" in her family affected what she said about herself and what she was willing to disclose to others who sought to help her. In this case and other cases where children's verbal communication is limited, some framework for understanding drawings may be necessary.

Looking with a "phenomenological eye" also includes accepting and expecting that each child has a different way of approaching art and an individual style of drawing with particular likes or dislikes for colors, forms, and compositions in their art expression. Children, like adults, have preferences for colors, certain images they like to draw, compositional styles and other characteristics that they may repeatedly use in their work. Mental health professionals, although perhaps not trained or experienced in visual art, also have preferences that may affect their understanding of children's work. Part of understanding children's drawings as unique phenomena includes understanding what you are personally attracted to in children's imagery, which images cause you to react strongly and which do not, and even realizing that you may reject or dislike some children's drawings. This esthetic response is part of how all individuals react to visual images, but for therapists who work with children's drawing, these responses become particularly important because these reactions do affect how drawings are judged, or which aspects are given attention.

CONCLUSION

To be meaningfully understood, children's drawings must be considered from a variety of contexts. Children draw for many reasons, some of which are uniquely related to their own developmental process, their affinity for drawing, and their personal experiences with art making. Although children bring their own unique thoughts, perceptions, and feelings into their creative work, their art expressions may also be influenced by the environment in which they draw or the materials with which they create. The impact of the therapeutic relationship is equally important, and issues of safety and trust as well as the therapist's enthusiasm, knowledge, and respect for the creative process can affect children's art expression both in areas of content and participation.

A phenomenological approach to understanding children's creative work is attractive because it entails looking at drawings from a variety of perspectives, including developmental, emotional, interpersonal, and other influences as well as taking into account the effect of materials, personal capacity for art expression, and therapeutic relationship. It makes possible the recognition that drawings can also be reflective of children's potentials, abilities, and capabilities. These are areas of strength, resilience, individuality, and personal heritage that contribute to the uniqueness of the individual child, and identifying these potentials is helpful in establishing an unbiased and integral understanding of children. This comprehensive awareness enables the counselor or therapist to communicate with children more effectively and sensitively and to develop sound intervention strategies.

There have been numerous studies and hypotheses about the meaning of children's drawings from various theoretical postions and philosophical slants. It is unfortunate that many of these studies reduce children's art expressions to lists of elements, such as details on houses, features or characteristics on human figures, or knotholes on trees. Although there may be certain meanings that can be assigned to the content of some drawings, what seems more beneficial and ethical is an appraisal of the many factors that affect how, what, and why children draw. When a therapist interprets a child's art expression without concern for the context in which the image was created, the clinician puts that child's expression "at risk" for misuse, misinterpretation, or misrepresentation. By adopting a more integral perspective, therapists reduce their own risk of misunderstanding the children whom they seek to serve and are more likely to be of greater help to children in general.

CHAPTER THREE

Working with Children and Their Drawings

This chapter suggests ways that therapists can work with children and their drawings. Because therapists as part of therapy are sometimes unfamiliar with the complexities of children's drawings, they may be inclined to judge children's artwork from limited experiences or viewpoints. Some prefer or are trained to use checklists of characteristics to interpret content while others react to a child's drawing as one would a photograph, seeing it for its literal qualities and missing its less tangible aspects. I believe, however, that therapists' need to explain images is genuine: When looking at the drawings of children who are in emotional pain, suffering from problems with their families, or reacting to extreme trauma or crisis, therapists want to relate their images to something occurring in these children's lives. The desire to find meaning and derive answers about children through their drawings is only natural, and even the most careful therapists often find themselves wanting to place significance on elements and content in the drawings of children, especially those children who are troubled, depressed, anxious, or fearful.

However, as already shown, interpreting children's creative work, whether from a list of characteristics such as those found in projective drawing literature or from one's own intuitive reactions, can be problematic. A simple example of how adults sometimes erroneously react to children's drawings is charmingly told by Antoine de Saint Exupéry in the story of *The Little Prince* (1943):

> Once when I was six years old I saw a magnificent picture in a book about the primeval forest. It was a picture of a boa constrictor in the act of swallowing an animal. . . . In the book it said: "Boa constrictors swallow their prey whole, without chewing it." . . . After some work with a

colored pencil I succeeded in making my first drawing [Figure 3.1]. I showed my masterpiece to the grown-ups, and asked them whether the drawing frightened them. But they answered: "Frighten? Why should any one be frightened by a hat?" (pp. 3–4)

Although the story's narrator goes on to add details to make a second drawing (Figure 3.2) showing the boa constrictor with the contents visible to the viewer (an X-ray drawing), adults who saw the drawing continued to respond incorrectly to his artwork. Eventually, he decided sadly not to draw again because he was continually misunderstood. This scenario, charmingly told by de Saint Exupéry, is common among therapists who look at children's art expressions with preconceived notions or narrow frameworks, not understanding that there is often more to children's drawings than meets the eye.

This excerpt also underscores an important point in understanding and responding to children's drawings: It is difficult for adults to see children's drawings with anything but their own adult eyes. It is hard to remember the imagination, creativity, and lack of rules that children have about art expression and often, in responding to their work, it is easy to be judgmental rather than open to many diverse possibilities. For example, when a child uses his or her hands to make

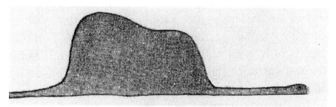

FIGURE 3.1. Drawing from The *Little Prince* by Antoine de Saint Exupéry. Copyright 1943 and renewed 1971 by Harcourt Brace & Company. Reprinted by permission.

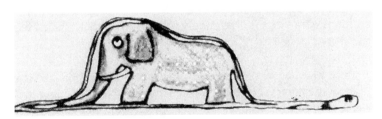

FIGURE 3.2. Drawing from *The Little Prince* by Antoine de Saint Exupéry. Copyright 1943 and renewed 1971 by Harcourt Brace & Company. Reprinted by permission.

lines in paint, what an adult may define as messy, a child may find enjoyable as play and as a sensory and kinesthetic experience. It is hard for adults to look at children's work, which is often colorful, visually compelling, and emotionally provocative, without imposing their own reactions and responses on it. It is important for therapists not to judge or interpret their drawings from adult standards and to attempt to understand not only the product of children's efforts but also what the process of drawing means to them.

DRAWINGS AS NARRATIVES

Drawings provide children with the potential to tell stories, convey metaphors, and present world views, both through what is present in the image itself and through their own responses to their images. The narrative qualities of children's drawings and children's interest in narrating them offer the therapist ways of understanding meaning from the child's perspective. A narrative, by definition, is a story or a recounting of past events, or a history, statement, report, account, description, or chronicle. By narrative qualities, I mean the ability of children's art expressions to present their impressions of their inner worlds, responses to their environments, and individual stories both through a developmentally appropriate form of communication (i.e., art) and through talking with the therapist about the content of their art expressions.

About children's art expressions as narratives, Riley (1997) writes:

> The therapist can step into the child's drawings and let him/her teach the meaning of this visual narrative. The art is a form of personal externalization, an extension of oneself, a visible projection of thoughts or feelings. When the art is accepted, honored, and validated by the therapist, the creator is (through identification with his/her product) equally accepted, honored, and validated. The client, in this case a child, can better understand through these actions than through words that he/she has been confirmed and valued. When the problem or anxiety has been externalized by the child in a drawing, it is the perfect time to confront the problem-laden behavior and still validate the worth of the creator (the child artist). (p. 2)

In recent years, therapists have come to view narratives as an important part of their work with clients, using clients' descriptions and stories about their lives, concerns, and world views to help them externalize problems (White & Epston, 1990). Narrative therapies have become increasingly popular in work with both children and their families (Freeman, Epston, & Lobovits, 1997), emphasizing regard for children's unique language, problem-solving resources, and perspectives. Many narrative therapists have realized the potential of art expression as a form of narrative with children. Since the goal of narrative therapy is to help to separate the problem or problem-laden behavior from the person through written narratives, I believe that art expression serves a similar narrative function for children by externalizing their experiences, thoughts, and feelings through visual images.

Like the narrative therapy approach, using drawing with children not only validates what they are experiencing and feeling, but also helps them to put some distance between themselves and their problems by making these tangible and visible. It is important in any therapeutic interaction with children to begin to establish that the *problem* is the problem, and that the child is not the problem, to paraphrase a well-known adage of narrative therapy (White & Epston, 1990). In my experience, drawing helps a great deal in establishing that the problem, whether it be a difficult feeling, behavior, or situation is separate from the self, by putting it out on paper.

A therapist using narrative approaches with children may rely largely on verbal storytelling to allow the child to share information about the content of his or her drawings, and with most children, this is helpful and necessary feedback about the meaning of their art expressions. However, it is also easy to see that for children, drawings themselves are an age-appropriate and effective form of narrative. Children do not have adult capabilities to articulate their emotions, perceptions, or beliefs verbally, and often, they prefer to convey ideas in ways other than talking. Many have noted the limits of using only verbal approaches with children (Axline, 1969; Case & Dalley, 1990; Gil, 1994; Malchiodi, 1990, 1997), highlighting the need for nonverbal forms of communication along with traditional talk therapy. The combination of both drawings and children's verbal descriptions provides therapists with an integrative means of understanding children. Drawings themselves not only allow children's narratives to emerge naturally, but permit the therapist to use these visual narratives as a way to interact with his or her child clients and can serve as a catalyst for children to communicate thoughts and concerns.

While one or two drawings may be helpful in understanding children and their visual and verbal narratives, in most cases, it is important to realize that this will often not be sufficient. Drawings are similar to freeze-frames: Each one presents a slightly different aspect of the child who makes them. Although there may be recurring themes, styles, or content in a child's drawings, each time a child creates a drawing, new images and details are often present. In seeing a series of drawings, witnessing the child's process in making drawings over time, and hearing several of the child's descriptions about his or her drawings, the therapist is given a more complete representation of the child.

PERSONAL BELIEFS ABOUT CHILDREN'S DRAWINGS AND THEIR USE IN THERAPY

Personal beliefs about children's drawings and their use in therapy are important to success in working with children and their art expressions. In order to identify one's personal beliefs about the role of drawing in therapeutic work, it is important for therapists first to formulate a goal for therapeutic work with drawings and children's communications about them. For some therapists, their goal may be to use drawings in assessment of children. Certainly, this is a common way in which drawings have been used in therapy with children for many years, particularly in the area of projective drawing tests and art-based assessments described earlier in this book. Other therapists may see drawing as an activity that helps children to work through emotional disturbance or traumatic experiences. In either case, it is vital to examine one's feelings about image making and one's views of the relative importance of drawing in the therapeutic process.

Because I have a background in visual art, I value the child's experience with the creative process of drawing, believing that it is important to allow and encourage the child to participate fully in art making in order for it to be effective and enjoyable. First, for drawing to be a positive, healing experience, the therapist must be convinced that the process of drawing helps the child to explore and transform conflicts and crises into healthy solutions, outlooks, and perspectives. This belief in the ameliorating aspects of creative activity within the safe container of the therapeutic relationship guides the child in working through problems and trauma through art expression.

Second, in order to make the experience a success, I believe that the person who asks or encourages children to draw must truly like art and the process of art making with children. Both the elements of play and an appreciation for images are intrinsic to success with drawings as therapeutic experiences with children.

Some questions that may help clarify one's beliefs include:

- Do you believe that drawing is a form of nonverbal communication in which the product is the most important element?
- Do you believe that drawing is also an important process through which change and transformation occur?
- How do you view the relative relationship between the process of drawing and the drawing itself (art product)? Is one more important than the other, or do both carry equal importance in therapy?
- How much time should be given to the activity of drawing and how much to talking with the child about the elements in the image?

By answering these questions, the helping professional can begin to clarify his or her perspectives and biases about the function and purpose of drawing in therapy.

THE ROLE OF THE THERAPIST IN THE DRAWING PROCESS

The presence of the therapist while the child is drawing is an important factor, particularly if the overall goal of using drawings is for a "curative" purpose, rather than solely for evaluation or assessment. In his many years of work with children, Allan (1988) notes that the presence of the therapist is an important factor, observing that "when a child draws in the presence of the therapist on a regular basis, then the healing potential is activated, conflicts expressed and resolved, and the therapist can gain a clearer and more accurate view of the conscious 'at work'" (p. 21). Clearly, as with any therapeutic alliance, the active presence of the helping professional is necessary for change to occur. I think it is important for the therapist to be in attendance, as a witness to the creative work, as a helper with materials and tasks, as a sustaining force in the creative process, and as safe receptacle for any powerful feelings that may arise either through the art or in conversation. The helping professional's presence maintains a "safe space" and the important healing factor of a positive interpersonal relationship between helping adult and child. By serving as the containing factor in the experience, the therapist provides a supportive and secure environment for children to experiment, play, and express themselves through art making.

In work with children who are troubled or traumatized, the very presence of the therapist can represent a nurturing, benevolent entity, one who offers the child a chance to express him- or herself with unconditional acceptance. Many disturbed children (and later on in life, disturbed adults) come to therapy or counseling because they have not experienced acceptance of themselves, particularly their creative abilities and self-expression. Being present during the drawing task is also extremely helpful in seeing how the child is doing with the task, allowing the therapist to intervene if necessary or to respond to any spontaneous conversation or questions the child may have.

Oddly enough, it takes some practice for some therapists to be able to sit patiently with a child and be present to the process of drawing. Some therapists feel uncomfortable watching a child draw and may feel the urge to walk away from the child while he or she is engrossed in drawing, fearing that they are viewed as intimidating or disruptive to the child's process. Some children are self-conscious and may not want the therapist to watch them, but in most cases, it is appropriate to be present during the activity. Therapists who are uneasy with drawing may find it difficult to be with children while they draw. Also, therapists' views of drawing in therapy may affect their interest or ability to be with children while they are drawing. If a therapist feels that the product is the only part of the drawing that is truly important, seeing it as an opportunity to analyze or interpret the elements in the image, then the process of drawing may hold little meaning. As previously mentioned, this is a limited way of working with children's drawings and may ignore the equally valuable process of the child and the relationship with the therapist during the drawing time.

Since drawing is a process, another important factor in working with children and their art expression is time. It is best to have enough time for children to work on their drawings and to allow them to become deeply involved in the process. Unfortunately, many therapy sessions today are limited to anywhere from 20 minutes to just under 1 hour, so children may not have enough time to complete drawings in some circumstances. It is necessary to convey to children how much time they have to do a task and when the session will end (in 5 minutes, 10 minutes, and so forth). Also, therapists themselves often feel rushed to get things accomplished, and it is important, if possible, not to transfer this feeling to children while they are drawing.

IS TALKING NECESSARY?

As already mentioned, one way of increasing understanding of the meaning of children's art expressions is to listen to children's narratives about their drawings. Simply asking children questions about their drawings encourages them to tell the therapist many things beyond the obvious visual content of the drawing itself. Like de Saint Exupery's story of his misinterpreted drawing, our understanding of children's drawings is often greatly enhanced by children's descriptions of them.

In my work with children, my personal goal through talking with them about their drawings is twofold: (1) to help the child externalize thoughts, feelings, events, and world views through artistic expression and storytelling; and (2) to help me to better understand the child's thoughts, feelings, and beliefs, and perceptions of events and the environment so that I can provide the best possible intervention on behalf of the child. While the latter goal focuses more on the area of assessment (i.e., evaluation of the child), for me, the first goal in working with children and their drawings is process-oriented.

Therapists who have not used drawings extensively in therapy with children often wonder if it is always necessary to have children talk about their drawings. In the course of my work with children, I have not interacted with many children who were unwilling to say something about their drawings. I believe that if the activity is appealing to a child, the therapeutic relationship is one of trust, and the environment is secure and supportive, the art process itself naturally leads to verbal communication and exchange. Engaging drawing naturally relaxes many children, allowing them to become absorbed in a creative and hopefully pleasurable task; by reducing some of the stress that brought them into therapy, they subsequently are more willing to talk with the therapist during or after drawing. For many children, drawing actually leads to wanting to share information that they might not otherwise disclose, especially if they feel comfortable with the creative activity or directive provided.

Although think it is important to have children say something about their art expressions, this may not always be possible, and once in a while, children may be resistant to talking about their drawings for various reasons. Some children may be shy or withdrawn, and some are just too young to talk. Children may also have language difficulties or speech problems, or English may not be their first language. Children who have been traumatized by abuse or violence may feel constricted when talking, especially if they have been threatened or told not to talk about themselves, their families, or their experiences (Malchiodi, 1990). Cultural background may influence some children who may have been taught by their parents to politely give short answers to questions and to limit interaction through speech or eye contact with adults in authority, and these cultural beliefs must be respected and accepted.

Fortunately, drawings themselves convey a great deal of information about children, the subject of the remainder of this book. However, because of what therapists can learn, I believe it is important for them to know how to talk to children about their drawings when this is appropriate. As delineated in the next section, a series of questions can be used to help therapists gather information about children's art products as well their process of drawing.

Talking during the Drawing Process

Therapists often wonder how much to talk with children while they are in the process of drawing. For standardized drawing tasks, usually no talking is allowed, although I often find myself breaking that rule if a child likes to talk to me while completing a drawing. With some children it is easy to see that they are engrossed in the activity and talking with them would be disruptive to what they are doing. Some therapists find it difficult not to talk and ask questions while the child is working and may even find it uncomfortable if the child does not respond verbally to the questions asked. Children may not respond for several reasons, one being that they are absorbed in the creative task at hand, wishing that the talkative adult would allow them to have full concentration on the drawing that the adult encouraged them to do in the first place. As Gardner (1982) noted in studies of young children, children even become annoyed by the adult who constantly interrupts the process by asking questions. For some children, any type of verbal disclosure may not be possible, particularly while trust in the therapeutic relationship is developing. However, there are also children who draw rather quickly, finish the task almost immediately, and want to talk about their work for a much longer time than it took to create it.

Other times, the therapist's questions may be problematic. For example, a question may be too probing for the stage of the therapeutic relationship, may be inappropriate, or the child may just not be able to answer it. Children who are fearful of revealing a family secret or those who have been abused often are not very verbally responsive to direct questions, particularly in the early stages of therapeutic work. Their art may say many things about the pain they are experiencing, but, as most therapists realize, children who are fearful of repercussions may be unwilling to talk at all in early stages. Many helping professionals who do not have very much experience or training in the use of drawing activities in therapy may actually encourage too much dialogue with the child, rather than allow the process of drawing to unfold.

Talking about the Finished Drawings

Because of their uncertainty about talking with children about their drawings, some therapists simply look at children's drawings for characteristics that may imply depression, trauma, or other feelings or perceptions and to make determinations about personality or development from these observations. However, through talking with children about their drawings, the therapist has the opportunity not only to learn more about the children with whom they work, but also to offer children the chance to express themselves and to grow through the process of creative activity within the framework of therapy.

In working with children's drawings, it is best to be judicious in the use and types of questions. Asking a child "why" he or she drew a particular element is usually unproductive. Most children have a difficult time explaining why they did something and will usually say in response that they "don't know" or may say nothing at all. In most situations, a more productive direction is to simply describe out loud what one sees in a drawing. For example, the therapist can refer to various elements in the drawing, saying, "I see a person looking out of the window of the house and a dog in the yard," or "I see a large yellow circle with blue wavy lines around it," waiting for a response from the child. Usually, the child will add some information about the picture, especially if the adult has missed some obvious feature or detail that is important to the child. The therapist can then continue to wonder out loud about the elements in the drawing, saying, perhaps, "I wonder what that person is thinking when he looks out of the window?" (waiting for the child to respond or comment); "I wonder what does he see when he looks out?"; or "I wonder what is the dog thinking?" (or feeling or doing, depending on the situation). As discussed earlier, this type of questioning implies taking a stance of "not knowing" on the part of the therapist and usually is effective in generating a productive conversation between therapist and child. In a real sense, one does not really know what an image means to the child, and by conveying one's interest in learning about the drawing in an open-ended way, the child is given the opportunity to explain elements in the drawing from his or her perspective.

The therapist's involvement in directing the course of activity and interaction is ultimately based on the therapist's own style of working with children. Solution-focused, cognitive-behavioral, or any number of other approaches may be taken. However, as in all therapeutic modalities with children, the clinician working with drawings will often reflect feelings back to the child, particularly when the child is obviously expressing powerful emotions in a drawing. Reflecting feelings back to the child helps to reinforce the therapist's acceptance of the content of the child's pictures and strengthens the natural process of the child in using drawings as reparation. For example, a 7-year-old boy who witnessed his mother being severely battered by his father drew a picture of his father (Figure 3.3) as a "bad man with a hammer and a knife" and said that he "was glad that he went to jail for what he did." The therapist might respond with "I guess seeing your dad hurt your mom really hurt you. It's OK not to like your dad because of what he did. I'm glad you are telling me about these feelings."

There are a number of general questions the therapist might ask a child at the completion of a drawing:

What title would you give this picture? Tell me about your drawing. Or, what is going on in this picture? These are broad questions that are helpful as openings to communication.

How do the people or animals in this picture feel? Since one of my goals in any therapeutic relationship with children is to help them to express feelings, I usually ask about the figures in the drawing, giving the child the opportunity to project or relate feelings through them. If there are objects (cars, houses, trees), the therapist might also ask how

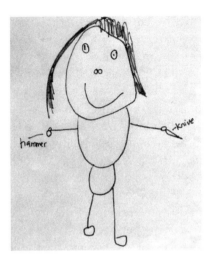

FIGURE 3.3. Drawing of a "bad man with a hammer and a knife" by a 7-year-old boy.

each of them feels. When I ask children about how inanimate objects feel, children may be confused (or think the therapist has a serious problem), so I often preface the question by saying that we are pretending that the house, car, or tree has feelings. If the drawing is composed of colors, shapes, or lines, the therapist may also ask "How does this shape (line or color) feel?"

How do the figures in the drawing feel about one another? If they could speak, what would they say to each other? These questions are related to expression of emotions, but they also may assist the child in developing a story about the drawing. The therapist may also pretend to be the voice of one of the figures, animals, or objects in the drawing and ask the child to speak for another figure in the drawing. This approach is similar to that of play therapy when using toys or sandtray figures in a dialogue with each other.

Can I ask the little girl, little boy, dog, cat, house, and so forth, something? Through this type of question, the child is encouraged to answer for the little girl, little boy, dog, cat, or house.

All of the questions discussed above are useful in generating a story about drawings. Most of the questions use a third-person approach rather than direct confrontation. Although many children will be quite comfortable in relating stories about their drawings from a first-person perspective, with some children, particularly those in therapy for serious trauma or disturbance, a more indirect approach to discussing drawings is useful. Using storytelling in the third person permits a degree of safety and distance and, at the same time, allows children to be the experts in relating meaning of their drawings.

Some children find it preferable to use a prop, such as a puppet, mask, or a toy to act out an answer to a question or to develop a story. As Oaklander (1978) notes, "It is often easier for a child to talk through a puppet than it is to say directly what he finds difficult to express. The puppet provides distance, and the child feels safer to reveal some of his innermost secrets this way" (p. 104). For example, the therapist might ask, "Would you like to use one these puppets (or masks) to talk? Can one of these toys answer the question I asked?" In my experience, talking with a child about drawings through a third person's voice by using either drawings or props such as puppets to explore images, naturally reduces feelings of shyness, anxiety, self-blame, guilt, and fear by creating a voice through which the child can safely speak.

For some children, drama or movement with or without props may be more appropriate and more enjoyable than purely drawing and talking. Sometimes I ask children to show me through movement what particular characters in their drawings would do if they could move or to help to dramatize the content of their art. Again, a set of puppets can also be used to act out a drawing through movement or to convey what might happen next in a drawing if the figures could move and talk.

A tape recorder can also encourage storytelling, with the added benefit of recording the story verbatim as it is told by the child. Most children like the playback feature, and it also allows me to comment or wonder out loud about other details of the story when we listen to it played back. The tape recorder can also be used as an interview device, especially if it has a microphone attachment; I have an older hand-held microphone that most children enjoy holding and speaking into. Even children who are quite shy get excited and animated. It works particularly well if the therapist can be a ham while doing the "interview."

MAKING SENSE OF THE DRAWING AND THE DRAWING PROCESS

In addition to asking children about their drawings, I use a series of questions to help me think about and understand their drawings. As discussed earlier, it is necessary for the therapist to consider both the process of drawing (how the child works with materials, experiences the session and activity, and interacts with the therapist) and the drawing itself. It is also important to recall the contextual nature of children's drawings in making observations; that is, it is vital to be aware of the effect of the environment and drawing materials on the drawing itself, and the impact of the therapeutic relationship (see Chapter 2).

It is also necessary to know how the child perceives the drawing task. For example, has he or she drawn spontaneously, or does the child see the drawing as a test? Many drawings created by children in therapy are spontaneous expressions or drawings children create for motives other than to satisfy a specific drawing protocol or assessment task. Therapists should be aware that children often recognize when they are being asked to make a drawing for the purpose of evaluation, at least in my experience. When a task is assigned to draw a house, tree, and a person with a pencil, for example, the child often suspects that this might be a test of some kind because the directions are specific, the theme is limited, and materials are restricted. On other occasions, children may see drawing as a creative activity, one that is experienced in school in an art class or session, rather than an intervention or a component of a treatment plan. Although therapists may be using drawing activities for their projective or treatment purposes, the child sees art in a different way and will hear a therapist's requests to make art with his or her own contextual understanding and from his or her own developmental perspective. The therapist's understanding of the child's perceptions of art making is an essential part of successful use of drawings in therapy and will enhance the therapeutic relationship by demonstrating the therapist's respect for the child's creative work.

I use the following questions when I am thinking about children's drawings and their process of drawing. There is no one correct or better answer to each these questions; they are not meant to have positive or negative implications about children, their responses to therapy, or their drawings. How a child responds will differ depending on the experiences of the individual child, the situation, the activity, and the interpersonal mix of therapist and child. These questions are offered merely as a way to help one organize observations and to review the child's responses to the session.

Process-related questions

- Does the child wait for directions or instruction, or is she or he impulsive about materials and beginning the drawing activity?
- Does the child seem calm and focused or restless and agitated? Active or withdrawn? Is the child able to concentrate, or does she or he appear distracted?
- Does this change during the session, with the art activity, or with any particular intervention or interaction?
- Is the child able to follow instructions, or is she or he easily frustrated or unable to follow simple instructions?
- Does the child seem confident in drawing or is she or he overly concerned about mistakes?
- Does the child seem to work independently or does she or he seem overly dependent on the therapist?
- To what degree does the child require structure or assistance in drawing?
- If in a group setting, can the child share materials and maintain appropriate boundaries?
- Does the child have difficulty leaving the session? How does the child respond to leaving her or his work if requested? Does the child seem excited to take the work with her or with him? Does the child specifically want the therapist to keep the drawing?

Product-related questions

- Is the child proud of the finished product, or does she or he devalue the drawing?
- Does the drawing contain unique expressive imagery, or does it contain stereotypic images?
- How does the child respond to questions about the drawing?
- Does the child associate images in the drawing with her- or himself, or does she or he not seem to self-associate with the drawing?
- Can the child discuss the drawing either metaphorically or in relationship to the self, or is discussing or describing the drawing difficult?
- Is the drawing developmentally appropriate for the child's age (see Chapter 4)?

With regard to product-related questions, some therapists may be looking for specific characteristics in drawings, in addition to the questions listed above. Again, it is important to remain open to the variety of meanings that children's images may have. Rather than focus solely on interpreting drawings, it is much more important in most situations to observe how children go about the assigned task, how they relate to the therapist, and how they respond to the drawings they have created.

When looking at a child's finished drawing I usually ask myself, "What seems unusual, emphasized, or important in the drawing?" and may use it as a point of conversation with the child. Such features or subjects can provide significant information about the child. A characteristic that is developmentally unusual is a good place to start (see Chapter 4). Remember, however, what is unusual or remarkable to adult eyes may just be part of normal developmental expression for a particular age or stage. For example, when a 6-year-old child draws a feature or object large, it may merely be the tendency of children at that age to emphasize something that is important to convey to the viewer. On the other hand, the child may be emphasizing something with color or lines because it represents something that is troubling or worrisome.

At the very least, noting what seems unusual in a drawing can provide an opening for conversation between therapist and child. For example, a 6-year-old girl was sent to me for evaluation and therapy because of suspected sexual abuse. After several drawings and getting to know each other, I asked her if she could draw me a picture of herself at home. She drew herself in her home, showing an X-ray view of her house with her in it. In the drawing there two floors drawn with many beds on the upper floor and a large coffee pot on the lower floor. The coffee pot struck me as interesting, so after I asked a couple of general questions about her drawing, I asked her about the coffee pot in the picture. She eagerly began to tell me about how everyone has a cup of coffee as they leave in the morning before they go to work. I asked her to name the people who had coffee before they left the house, and she named her mother and father and two older sisters who went to high school. When I asked who was left after that, she said that only she and her uncle, who was unemployed and who stayed home to watch her. The inclusion of the coffee pot in the drawing was an important piece of information that eventually confirmed that the uncle was sexually abusing the girl. It turned out to be a helpful element in letting the girl speak about her family and eventually provide clues to her sexual abuse.

RESISTANCE TO DRAWING

Some children have well-developed ideas about what they want to express and seem to have an intuitive sense about art making and their images. They need little or no direction from the therapist, are happy to create spontaneous images, and are content to have the therapist present as a catalyst, witness, and support for their work. However, children can, for various reasons, be resistant to drawing, even though they generally perceive it to be pleasant activity. Although there is no magic bullet to induce the resistant child to engage in drawing in therapy, there are some important factors involved in why some children might not draw and some ways to address the situation if it arises. In my own experience, I rarely find that children are resistant to drawing. I think that extensive experience in both art therapy and clinical counseling helps me to make the art process interesting and appealing to children. One intuitively knows what is exciting about art making, and children will get caught up in the therapist's enthusiasm.

In supervising therapists who use art activities with children, the question of resistance to drawing is one that frequently arises. If a therapist is more comfortable with verbal therapy and uncomfortable with art expression, art media, and the art process in children, this lack of confidence can affect the course of using drawing with children. Children will sense a lack of enthusiasm or skill in using art for either therapy or communication and, in response, will lose their enthusiasm and level of involvement in the process. For therapists with less experience in art or art therapy, asking children to draw may not automatically give the desired results.

The art supplies provided may inadvertently create resistance, too. As mentioned in Chapter 2, it is important to provide good quality materials with which to draw and high-quality paper to draw on. Markers that are dried out, crayons that are old and broken, paper that tears easily, or lack of a full range of colors can be not only discouraging but also frustrating to children. In order to engage a child in drawing, drawing materials that are in good shape and are visually exciting to use will go a long way to encourage children to engage in art making and self-expression.

Some children will be resistant to drawing for other more personal reasons, including worry, mistrust, or depression. Some children are so highly defended and fearful it is sometimes impossible for them to draw; being expressive through drawing is perceived as threatening and anxiety-producing. Sometimes the task itself creates the resistance; for example, asking a child who does not feel safe or protected within the therapeutic relationship to draw a traumatic experience or assigning a child with family problems a family drawing in the early stages of treatment can be a threatening experience.

There are a few approaches one can try to help overcome resistance. Sometimes I begin the drawing for the child, asking the child for directions as to content, form, or other characteristics. Although I started out my professional life as an artist and have some degree of skill in drawing, sometimes it actually is helpful not to be skilled artistically. A bit of fumbling can induce the child to want to get involved and to correct the therapist's inaccuracies or lack of skill. One can even draw primitive stick figures and suddenly find that a child is adding details or "improving" upon the drawing.

With really resistant children, I play a cartoon game in which I am the cartoonist who draws whatever the child would like me to draw. I might start the cartoon strip with an image such as Garfield (one character I know how to draw) and then ask the child to tell me what the character is doing. Usually, one of two things happens: The child becomes intrigued with dictating a story for me to draw, thus providing a plot I can add to or help the child develop or problem solve. Some children get immediately interested in the cartoon process (especially if I am inept in recreating the characters) and take over drawing the cartoon. One can also switch back and forth between child and therapist, each drawing one frame of the cartoon at a time.

Sometimes what seems like resistance to drawing may only be insecurity about the situation or a lack of confidence in how and where to begin. Providing a child with a large piece of white paper and drawing materials with the assignment of "draw anything you want" can be overwhelming, especially with children who are fearful, anxious, or unsure of themselves. At other times children need a warm-up to get them started and to establish the confidence and trust necessary to feeling safe to express. Asking the child to pick one detail of what she or he was planning to draw may be helpful. For example, if the child is drawing a human figure, the therapist might ask if she or he could simply draw the head. From that point, the child could be encouraged to draw other features such as eyes, nose, and mouth, a body, legs, and so forth. Often once engaged in the process, the child will continue with little prompting.

Steele (1997) has developed a simple technique that could be used to stimulate children who are resistant to drawing for whatever reason. He asks the child to make a thumb print on an index card (the size is important here, since a small index card is less threatening than a large piece of paper for some children) and to add details to it to create a special friend or companion. The thumb print becomes a spontaneous way to motivate children to draw an image of a figure. This figure could easily become the central figure in a larger drawing with additional elements such as a house, other people, or animals.

Lastly, showing other children's drawings or simple images may be helpful, especially with children who are insecure about their abilities. Some children may try to copy the drawings, but usually they soon begin to put their own images into their drawings or change the images in more personal ways. The Silver Drawing Test (1996a) pictures (a series of simple line drawings of various people, animals, and objects) have come in handy from time to time to stimulate children who feel they cannot think of anything to draw or feel too insecure about creating their own images. Silver's cards are also particularly good with children who may not have the energy to draw, such as physically ill children in the hospital for surgery or treatment. The child can simply choose two or three cards and arrange them to tell a story to the therapist. The child can also copy the images and change them in whatever way he or she wants.

It is important to note that there are some children who will comply with the therapist's requests to draw even when drawing may not be the most productive means of expression for them. Some may be more suited to a different form of art expression, such as collage or clay work, and others may be more expressive through media such as puppets, drama, play, or movement. While most children will engage in drawing, the therapist has to be sensitive to what modality, whether art, movement, play, or verbal storytelling, is most conducive to engaging them in therapy and getting children to express themselves freely.

RESPONDING TO SEXUAL OR VIOLENT CONTENT IN CHILDREN'S DRAWINGS

In supervisory sessions with mental health professionals, I am frequently asked about sexual or violent content in children's drawings (see Chapter 5). Many therapists, even those who have worked with children for many years, are understandably uncomfortable with or even frightened by drawings that contain explicitly sexual or violent material. When therapists use art expression as a way for children to communicate thoughts, feelings, and ideas that children may not openly discuss, sexual or violent content that is difficult to express through words may appear in drawings. Therapists have to be prepared to accept and respond to these powerful and often overwhelming images. It may be more comfortable for a helping professional to see stereotypic hearts, rainbows, and smiling faces rather than blatantly sexual or violent content. However, powerful affect in drawings should not be discouraged just because the therapist is uncomfortable with it.

When I first started work as an art therapist many years ago, I was conducting an evaluation of a 13-year-old boy who presented me with a somewhat shocking human figure drawing (Figure 3.4) at our first meeting. He was referred to me to assess and treat his behavioral problems, hyperactivity, and learning disabilities as part of a special program at his public school. The boy had some moderate learning disabilities in the area of reading and language, was diagnosed by the school psychologist as having what is now known as attention-deficit\hyperactivity disorder (ADHD) and often behaved immaturely, having little self-control over his behavior in the classroom and with peers. We were to meet for weekly art therapy sessions for the semester at his school in his special classroom.

What is obviously shocking about the drawing are the highly sexual features. Although the boy was a preadolescent, capable of realistic drawings, nudity and emphasized sexual characteristics are unusual details for this age group. The boy's affect after completing the drawing was mixed; he laughed uncontrollably at first (probably at my shocked face), then suddenly seemed disturbed and ashamed of his drawing. I asked him who the person in this drawing was and he quietly said "me" and would say no more at that time. This drawing began a series of art therapy sessions to address the content presented in the drawing, including the sexual content and his feelings about himself. Unfortunately, in this boy's case, he had been sexually and physically abused by his father and felt abandoned by his mother who did not report or protect him from his father's abuse.

Being a novice therapist at the time, I was quite surprised to receive this image from the boy. Since then, I have seen a great many drawings with overtly sexual content, most of them from children who have been sexually abused. Therapists who work with children

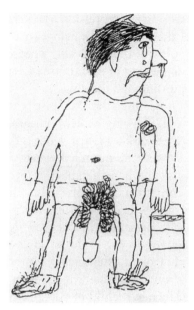

FIGURE 3.4. Pencil drawing of a person by a 13-year-old boy.

who have been sexually abused in some way are obviously likely to see a great deal of images that have overtly sexual content. Some of these images may be disturbing depending on the therapist's past experiences and feelings about sexual images. While it is natural to be shocked by these images, the therapist must examine how he or she reacts to this type of imagery because personal reactions to sexual content will affect how one interacts with the child and the child's drawing. Supervision from a therapist with expertise in understanding children's drawings or simply from another peer professional can be very useful to eliminate blindspots in one's thinking and observations concerning disturbing, violent, or sexual imagery. Live or video supervision of the therapist interacting with children is also extremely helpful, particularly in learning interview skills and one's responses to children's art activities (Malchiodi & Riley, 1996).

In some ways, violent imagery in drawings can be even more problematic and is equally difficult to confront. Although some young children draw images that contain obviously violent content, older children and adolescents are more likely to draw pictures that may have violent or frightening images. Some of these drawings come from children and adolescents who have been abused and are either reenacting the abuse or using art expression as a vehicle to act out feelings or wishes to hurt their abusers. Drawings that depict violent content directed at the self or others are also worrisome, particularly if there is concern for depression or suicide (see Chapter 5 for a discussion of childhood depression and drawings).

Haeseler (1987) notes that the therapist "can help patients understand their intent in drawing violent images—do they wish to shock others, punish them, ask for help? What is the timing and manner of presentation? Who is the intended viewer?" (p. 15). These are basic questions to consider when therapists are working with and responding to violent content in drawings. Also, therapists can be accepting of the violent content in a drawing but not accepting of the behavior or violent act represented in the drawing. This is an important distinction to convey to the child or adolescent who creates a drawing with obviously violent or upsetting content. As in any therapeutic relationship or situation, safety is a paramount issue and one that must be addressed when a child or adolescent draws images that convey violent or cruel themes.

Graham (1994) in his work with emotionally disturbed adolescents describes several reasons why teenagers make drawings with violent imagery:

> a) it usually guarantees responses; b) it can be shocking, and in eliciting an emotional response from the viewer, it substantiates the artist's power as a maker of images that is thrilling to the artist; and c) it is a way to distinguish the artist from others in a way that response to beauty cannot. The beholder of beauty feels transcendent and the art seems without author; when we see shocking art, we may recoil, but we soon ask "Who did it?" and "Why?" (p. 118)

Unfortunately, many children who are in extreme emotional pain or are severely depressed will resort to stereotypes to avoid expressing or communicating the real issues that are troubling their lives. Drawings with violent themes are not only visually compelling and shocking, but often much more revealing of specific problems and feelings a child is experiencing. Violent images, although perhaps offensive and disturbing to the therapist, convey important responses and for some children and adolescents may even be a way to translate violent thoughts or wishes into a more acceptable form.

CONCLUSION

This chapter has presented a brief overview of considerations and ways to work with children through their drawings. As mentioned in the beginning of this chapter, therapists often react to children's drawings from their own perspective, but by asking appropriate questions, children's narratives about their art expressions can often enhance understanding. Examining one's personal beliefs about drawing and its meaning in therapy with children can also be helpful in working with children. As with any therapeutic technique, the use of drawings in therapy requires feedback, not only for difficult cases, but to keep a check on biases one may have about the content of art expressions.

In working with children and their drawings, it is always helpful to keep in mind the goal of using drawings with children in therapy. Steele (1997), reflecting on many years of working with traumatized and grieving children, notes:

> Your [the therapist's] function in the drawing process is to encourage the child to draw about his experience and tell his story. In the process, he finds relief from his terror while giving you a better "picture" of what that terror is like for him. It is a process that encourages a renewed sense of inner control and empowerment. Simply by being curious and inquisitive about what he draws, you provide the vehicle and opportunity he needs to diminish the power of those terrifying sensory memories and replace them with more positive pleasurable memories. (p. 43)

It is important for therapists to remember that, through drawing, children allow them into their inner world of experiences, sharing as well as exposing themselves. While children's drawings convey information about their feelings, thoughts and fantasies, it is the process of drawing and the active presence of the therapist interacting with the child that encourage reparation and recovery through creative activity.

CHAPTER FOUR

Developmental Aspects of Children's Drawings

The intriguing fact that most children go through a predictable sequence of artistic expression is essential to understanding all other aspects of children's drawings. After more than 20 years of working and observing children making art, I am still fascinated by the idea that all children, barring severe handicapping conditions, are compelled to make scribbles at young ages, are eventually able to visually represent human forms and objects, and are capable of combining these elements in drawings with themes and personal meaning. In short, throughout childhood, all children follow expected, progressive changes in their drawing, changes that are characteristic of each age group. These stages of artistic development appear to be universal to children throughout the world, commonalities of mark-making that are part of every normal child's ability to communicate through art expression.

One could easily fill several volumes with all the material that has been written on children's artistic development. Although there are many detailed discussions about the developmental stages of children's art, many therapists have at best a very simple working knowledge of how normal children draw at various ages, and others are totally unfamiliar with the theory of developmental stages in artistic expression. Knowing how children normally express themselves through drawing at various ages is essential to understanding children's drawings in general. This foundation gives therapists a point of comparison that is particularly useful when working with children with cognitive, developmental, or physical problems, and those who have experienced trauma, crisis, or emotional disturbance in their lives.

This chapter does not intend to replace the many comprehensive texts available on children's artistic development. I have attempted, however, to condense the most basic and salient information on normal stages for those readers who may not be familiar with the stages of artistic development and who need a foundation for initial understanding. This fundamental information covers what most therapists and others who work with children need to know in order to effectively understand developmental aspects of children's drawings. Additional suggestions for further study and information are found throughout this chapter and in the reference section at the end of the book.

DEVELOPMENTAL LEVELS IN CHILDREN'S ART

In the late 1800s and early 20th century, researchers interested in children's artistic expression began to describe the stages observed in drawing development. This early work concluded that children go through three general stages of artistic development:

1. A *scribbling stage*, which consists of both unsystematically scattered lines and later scribbling in the form of clustered lines and circular shapes.
2. A *schematic stage* in which children develop schemata to represent human figures, objects, and environments.
3. A *naturalistic stage* in which there are more realistic, lifelike details.

This preliminary work, although broad and general, served as the catalyst for more specific analyses and the eventual establishment of more detailed information on stages of drawing development. As early as 1921, Burt studied and classified children's drawings into several distinct stages. He observed that children begin making scribbles at the age of 2 to 3 years, old, and by age 4, single lines emerge, setting the stage for creating basic forms representing people and animals. By age 5 or 6 years, he concluded, children are able to draw forms that represent things they see in their environments, and from 7 to 11 years, children increase in their abilities to portray objects and figures realistically with the discovery of spatial depth, motion, and color in nature. Burt noted that children tend to discard art in preadolescent years, repressing their interest in art expression either because of lack of confidence in abilities or lack of encouragement from others. Goodenough (1926; see Chapter 1) also observed a developmental sequence of artistic expression and attempted to establish age norms through the analysis of children's drawings with the goal of creating a measure of intelligence.

Subsequently, others have observed a sequential pattern in children's art and have arrived at theories of artistic development in children. Possibly the most well-known is the work of Lowenfeld (1947), the author of a comprehensive text on children's artistic expressions, *Creative and Mental Growth*; his original work was later updated and some material eliminated after his death in several revised editions (Lowenfeld & Brittain, 1982). Many art educators and therapists still use Lowenfeld's stages as a standard for assessing artistic development in children, particularly in the field of art therapy.

Lowenfeld believed that children's growth through art was analogous to the process of organizing thoughts and the development of cognitive abilities. In this sense, art expressions are indications of children's emerging abilities in many areas—motor skills, perception, language, symbol formation, sensory awareness, and spatial orientation. Lowenfeld based his ideas on much of the earlier work of Burt and others, describing six major stages of artistic development:

1. *Scribbling* (ages 2 to 4 years): earliest drawings often kinesthetically based, eventually becoming representative of mental activity; various types of scribbles including disordered, longitudinal, and circular; naming of scribbles at the end of this stage.
2. *Preschematic* (ages 4 to 7 years): early development of representational symbols, particularly rudimentary forms representing humans.
3. *Schematic* (ages 7 to 9 years): continuing development of representational symbols, particularly a schema for figures, objects, composition, and color; use of a baseline.
4. *Dawning realism* (ages 9 to 11 years): increasing skill at depicting spatial depth and color in nature, along with increasing rigidity in art expression.
5. *Pseudorealism* (ages 11 to 13 years): more critical awareness of human figures and environment and increasing detail; increasing rigidity in art expression; caricature.
6. *Period of decision* (adolescence): expression is more sophisti-

cated and detailed; some children do not reach this stage unless they continue or are encouraged to make art.

Others have continued to explore children's artistic development, adding not only to the overall knowledge of developmental
characteristics of art activities from very young children through adolescence but also providing divergent viewpoints on the process of
artistic development. For example, Pasto (1965) considers children's
art expressions not only from a development lens but also as emotional experiences in what he terms his "space–frame" theory. He makes
suggestions about the symbolism of various forms during early art expression, such as children's first attempts at drawing circles as representations of mother images and rectangles as symbols of forming
identity separate from the rest of the world. These observations seem
to draw from Jungian and other psychological theories of the time,
rather than solely human development models, offering an additional
framework for understanding emotional growth and maturation.

Winner (1982), Golomb (1990), and Gardner (1980) provide
more thoroughly researched concepts for understanding children's
drawings from the perspectives of developmental psychology, art, and
to some extent, anthropology. Gardner offers a similar descriptive set
of stages to that of Lowenfeld, including scribbles, early forms, development of first human figures, schematic representations, realism,
preadolescent caricatures, and adolescent artistic abilities. Gardner
(1980), like others, agrees that young children throughout the world
appear to go through specific, predictable stages of artistic development, beginning at an early age and continuing through adolescence.

Although various names have been given to stages of artistic expression, for the sake of clarity in this text they are defined as follows:
Stage I: scribbling; Stage II: basic forms, Stage III: human forms and
beginning schemata; Stage IV: development of a visual schema, Stage
V: realism; and Stage VI: adolescence. The major landmarks of each
stage are condensed and highlight the important aspects of that stage.
Age ranges given are approximate; in other words, there may be some
overlap in ages, drawing style, skills that may still be considered normal expression at a given stage. It is also important to remember that
children may also go back and forth between stages. For example, a
child in Stage III may draw human figures one day and make less complex forms typical of Stage II the next. This type of fluctuation is common and to be expected in all children.

For mental health professionals who are familiar with Piaget's studies of children's intellectual growth (Piaget, 1959; Piaget & Inhelder, 1971), it may be helpful to know that the stages of artistic development described in this chapter roughly correspond to his theory of cognitive development. The scribbling stage (Stage I) parallels the latter part of the sensorimotor period, and the two stages following it, basic forms (Stage II) and human forms and early schemata (Stage III) could be considered part of the preoperational period which lasts up until approximately age 7. In Piaget's outline, a period of concrete operations follow from ages 7 to 12, which parallels the emergence of a visual schema (Stage IV) and interest in realistic drawing (Stage V). Lastly, the final period, usually called formal operations and thought to begin at 12 years, coincides with adolescent artistic development (Stage VI). References to this theory of cognitive development are briefly included throughout this chapter to help the reader make connections between children's cognitive development and their artistic development.

For therapists who use drawings with children occasionally, this brief section should provide you with a basic foundation in understanding art expressions from a developmental point of view. For those therapists who regularly use drawings with children in treatment and assessment, a more in-depth review of the material mentioned in this chapter is probably necessary. When in doubt, a consultation with an experienced art therapist, art educator, or child development specialist may be needed.

Stage I: Scribbling

This first stage occurs in children from approximately ages 18 months to 3 years and is a time when the very first marks are made on paper (or on walls, in books, or other inappropriate surfaces, if the child is not supervised). As previously noted, this stage of artistic development coincides with the latter part of the sensorimotor period of cognitive development (Piaget, 1959; Piaget & Inhelder, 1971) and, to some extent, the beginning of preoperational thinking. In terms of sensorimotor experiences, this is the time of a child's life when he or she thinks kinesthetically, begins to improve eye–hand coordination, and starts to climb, walk, and run. There is a gradual development of goal-directed, purposeful behavior, and children often delight in imitating the speech and actions of others around them. Toward the end of this stage (age 3 years), symbolic thinking begins and children start to classify what they see in their environment by form, color, and size. The development of language also plays an increasingly important role.

The first scribble drawings a child makes at ages 1½ to 2 years are spontaneous in that no one teaches a very young child how to scribble. At first there is little control of the motions that are used to make the scribble; in fact, very young children are as likely to chew on the crayon as to scribble with it. Accidental results occur, and the line quality of these early drawings varies greatly (Figures 4.1–4.3).

Scribbling and other early drawing activities have been related to kinesthetic experiences and to practicing coordination between visual and motor activity. To some extent, this is true in that young children are practicing and developing articulation of gross and eventually fine motor control. However, interestingly enough, children do know that they are making marks and enjoy the experience of putting crayon to paper. Gonas and Yonas (in Winner, 1982) note that if you replace a

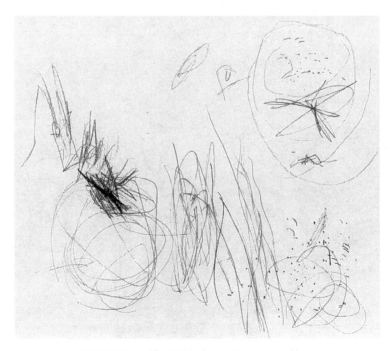

FIGURE 4.1. Scribble drawing by a 2-year-old girl.

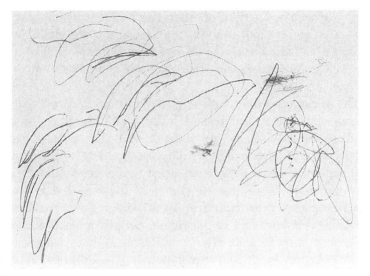

FIGURE 4.2. Scribble drawing by a 2-year-old girl.

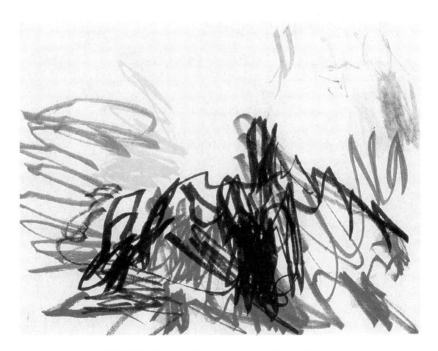

FIGURE 4.3. Scribble drawing by a 3-year-old boy.

child's marker with one that leaves no trace, a child will stop scribbling. So although children enjoy the movement of their arms, they are also intrigued with the process of making a mark on paper or other surface.

There are various theories as to the meanings of scribbles, partly because it is hard to attribute meaning to them. Early researchers have noted that scribbles are unintentional mark-making that merely record movements of the arm, wrist, and hand (Burt, 1921; Goodenough, 1926). However, that observation has changed in recent decades. Although a child's scribble drawing may look like a meaningless snarl of lines to an adult, the child who creates one is also developing in the ability to express him- or herself in language and gestures. This suggests that scribbles may also have meaning in that they may represent something to the child, although not necessarily a pictorial representation. For example, what looks like random lines may represent a dog running or a balloon floating, depicting a gesture that symbolizes a motion rather than a literal picture of the object. Scribbles are children's awakenings to the concept that lines and shapes on paper can also represent things in their environment.

Adults who watch children scribble may also play a role in the development of meanings in these early drawings. Observing adults often suggest that scribbles stand for people, animals, or objects, asking, "Are you drawing a picture of Daddy?" or "Is that your cat?" Children may come to realize that others expect their scribbles to represent something, or the scribbles may accidentally look like people, animals, or trees, and the child may connect ideas with mark-making activities.

There have been various attempts to categorize scribble drawings. Lowenfeld (1947) for example, classified children's scribbles into four stages: (1) disordered, implying no control of motions and often appearing chaotic and disorganized; (2) longitudinal, implying repeated motions and the establishment of some coordination and control of mark-making; (3) circular, describing even greater control in that additional motor skills and complexity are required; and (4) naming scribbles, which Lowenfeld believed to be a change from kinesthetic to imaginative thinking in the child. In other words, as children's motor skills progress, they begin to form repeated motions with their scribbles, making horizontal or longitudinal lines, circular shapes, and assorted dots, marks, and other forms. There is no intentional use of line by the child at this age to make representational marks or symbolic forms. At this stage there is also not much conscious use of color (i.e., the color is used for enjoyment without specific intentions), and children are often unconcerned with color choice, producing a series of scribble drawings without changing crayons. Drawing is also enjoyed for the kinesthetic experience it provides.

Gardner (1980) mentions some additional types of scribble "behavior" including dots and jabs, and writing forms. These are somewhat similar to Lowenfeld's observations, but focus more on defining the process of scribbling. Dots and jabs are staccato-like movements of drawing instrument to paper, often mixed in with other types of scribbles (see Figure 4.2). For example, scribbles Gardner calls "writing forms" are thought by him to be children's attempts to mimic adult signatures (Figure 4.4) and may serve as early practice runs in developing abilities to print and write one's own name.

Rhoda Kellogg (1969) has conducted some of the most extensive research on children's early graphic activity and considers scribble pictures important to the development of more advanced art expression. She proposes that children go through a progressive sequence of scribbling that starts with simple marks and eventually becomes more com-

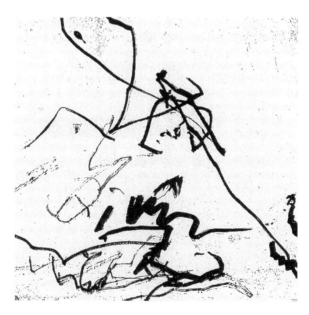

FIGURE 4.4. Scribble drawing by a 2½-year-old boy that includes lines resembling signatures and handwriting.

plex patterns and designs. Kellogg documented this sequence (1969) through analyzing children's scribbles between the ages of 2 and 3, arriving at 20 basic scribbles that are the foundation for later graphic development (Figure 4.5). Golomb (1981, 1990) later simplified Kellogg's observations to two types of scribbles—loops and circles (circular movement), and parallel lines (horizontal, vertical, or diagonal movement).

Although it is interesting to think about the variety of scribble forms that children produce, it is probably not really important for the average therapist to know all the names of scribble types and styles that have been coined through adult eyes. What is important to understand is the developmental significance of this stage, why children

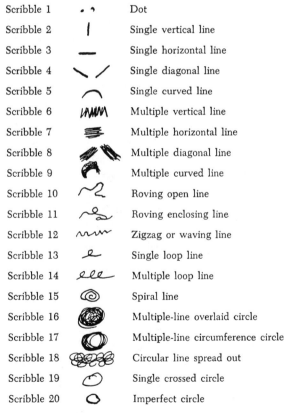

FIGURE 4.5. Twenty basic scribbles according to Kellogg. From *Analyzing Children's Art* by Rhoda Kellogg. Copyright 1970 by Rhoda Kellogg. Reprinted by permission of Mayfield Publishing Company.

experience it, and how it impacts later artistic development. Whichever author's classification is used, it is obvious that these first marks on paper are the foundations for later drawings and early experimentation with lines and shapes through scribbling is important to later progress.

Finally, children at the ages of 2 and 3 years may begin to use the space of the paper in various ways, indicating a recognition of the edge of the paper. They may begin to place lines and marks in various ways or placements. Kellogg (1969) identified 17 of these placement patterns, noting that children also begin to create shapes such as triangles or rectangles in the clustered lines (Figure 4.6). By about 3 years (Stage II), children begin drawing these shapes with a single line instead of a group of scribbled lines.

In addition to the developmental characteristics of children's drawings at this age, there are some additional important considerations for therapists who use art with very young children. First and foremost, young children have a limited attention span and limited motor skills for art activities. There also is not much content other than scribbled lines, and there is not likely to be much narrative from the child concerning the art product (except in the latter part of this stage and the proceeding one in which children begin to name and talk about their scribbles in imaginative ways). However, it is still important to provide the opportunity for young children at this age to draw, because most will enjoy the purely expressive and movement qualities of the experience. It is also meaningful to observe if the child feels comfortable with drawing through scribbling, as children who may have some developmental or even emotional difficulty may not be at ease with expressing themselves in this way.

Stage II: Basic Forms

From ages 3 to 4 years, children may still make scribbles, but they also become even more involved in naming and inventing stories about them. This stage of artistic development roughly parallels the early part of the preoperational period, particularly the preconceptual phase lasting from two to four years (Piaget, 1959). During this phase of cognitive development, children are considered to be egocentric and begin to have at least a subjective notion of cause and effect. As previously noted, there is an increasing importance of language, symbolic

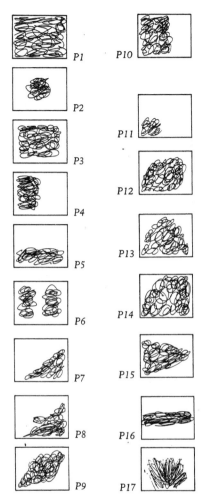

FIGURE 4.6. Scribble placement patterns according to Kellogg. From *Analyzing Children's Art* by Rhoda Kellogg. Copyright 1970 by Rhoda Kellogg. Reprinted by permission of Mayfield Publishing Company.

thought is emerging, and children can classify their world through form, color, and size.

Scribbles and other artistic expressions made during this stage signal a developmental landmark, since now children can connect their motions and marks on paper to the world around them. Because narratives about drawings become more important by this age, it is valuable for therapists to know that children will actively seek to talk about their drawings, even if they appear to adults as unidentifiable scribbles. However, as an observing adult you may see very little resemblance in the drawing to what the child is meticulously telling you in his or her story.

Gardner (1980) has explored this phenomenon of "romancing" or naming the scribbled image extensively, concluding that there is no simple explanation for the descriptions that children give about their scribbles. If adults are asking children about their drawings, it may be likely that in order to please them, children simply tell them a story about the image. On the other hand, since it is difficult to see through the eyes of the child artist, he or she may be genuinely making marks that have some sort of meaning and may be moving forward in his or her development of representational images. Also, to complicate our understanding, naming of scribbles occurs frequently with some young children and sometimes not at all or rarely with others.

The stage is significant for therapists working with children in that storytelling can now be introduced as a component of art making. Conceivably, a child might tell the listening adult something important through talking about a scribble, but the situation also is problematic, since children of this age may still not be very attentive to the drawing task for long periods of time because of limited attention spans. Storytelling may be difficult at best because young children's vocabularies are limited in scope, and their concentration is restricted. Also, be aware that the content of scribble drawings varies greatly, and narratives may change substantially even over the course of several minutes. A child may start a scribble drawing by saying, "This is my mommy," only to quickly label the figure as something else soon after. In fact, the next day the child may rename the drawing yet again, identifying it as something completely different; the day after that the scribble drawing may mean something else again.

For example, Catelin, a 3½-year-old girl made a scribble drawing with felt markers (Figure 4.7) a few minutes after her grandmother reprimanded her for spilling her juice and cookies on the floor outside the art and play room. When I asked Catelin for a title for her picture, she said it the "black bug monster who yells at her for doing bad things," an obvious reference to the incident with her grandmother moments before and perhaps a reference to other times when she had been punished or scolded. The scribble has very controlled repetition of short lines, larger movements of lines across half the paper, and some forms consisting of wider lines; since Catelin was obviously an-

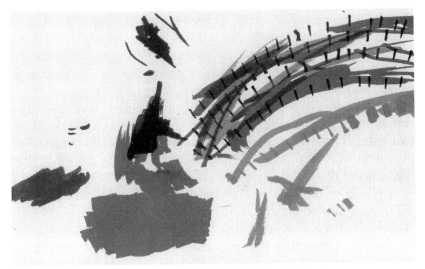

FIGURE 4.7. Scribble drawing by 3-year-old Catelin.

gry and upset when she came into the session that day, I imagine the line qualities of her drawing reflected her feelings. However, the next day when Catelin came back to the art room and looked at her picture, she said it was about music, renaming it "Catelin's Music," and when asked, she had no recall of the "black bug monster" of the previous day. This is normal for children of this age, and therapists should be aware that changing meaning of visual symbols is appropriate at this stage in drawing development.

Gardner (1980) makes one other important point about naming scribbles, identifying two types of behaviors in young children that may be significant to understanding their drawings and communications about their images. He observed two types of responses to both the process of scribble-making and talking about scribble images. Some children are "patterners"; that is, they are interested in patterns, and characteristics such as colors, size, and shape. They enjoy exploration and experimentation but often are not particularly interested in social interaction. Other children may be what Gardner (1980) calls "dramatists." They tend to be more interested in actions and adventures, and dramatic stories and tales. These children like to pretend through storytelling and enjoy social contact with peers and adults. Both patterners and dramatists seem to like to draw, but patterners tend not to make comments about their images unless prompted in order to quiet inquisitive adults. Dramatists, on the other hand, find talking about the image as exciting as making the image, as well as relating real or imagined stories to listening adults. There may also be children who do not neatly fit into either category or who may seem to fluctuate between the two styles.

Although Gardner's study (1980) of patterners and dramatists was derived from observations of a small number of children, these two styles of interacting with art expressions are important for therapists who work with children and their drawings to consider. Play therapists or those clinicians who use therapeutic play in the form of storytelling or dramatic enactment may find some children (the dramatists) more eager and more able to express themselves through action-oriented modalities. Other children may enjoy becoming more involved in constructing drawings and prefer to enjoy the activity for what it is, rather than reenacting it or talking about it extensively. While I am not advocating that therapists assess and label children as either patterners or dramatists, it is important for therapists to be sensitive to children's preferences in art-making activity at this stage when children exhibit these types of propensities for creative work.

In addition to scribbles, more complex configurations emerge at this time: mandalas (circular shapes, designs, or patterns) and shapes such as triangles, circles, crosses, squares, and rectangles (Kellogg, 1969). For children these are elements that provide practice for the development of more representational pictures in the near future. During this stage, the normal child's visual language is rapidly developing to include the basic forms needed to make human figures and other forms, the main milestone in the next stage of artistic development.

Kellogg notes that, when mandalas begin to appear, they often include a combination of a cross and a circle, square or rectangle (Figure 4.8). The mandala in both child and adult art has received a great deal of attention and speculation from many sources in art, anthropology, and psychology. Many authors have noted mandalas in children's drawings as well as in adult drawings in many cultures (Jung, 1960; J. Kellogg, 1993). Jung believed that the mandala constituted an archetypal image of the collective unconscious, symbolizing balance and harmony. Although Rhoda Kellogg agreed, she also observed that the mandala recapitulates and combines the previous shapes and lines that children have learned how to make. Allan (1988) notes that "Mandalas reflect the development of protective walls which function

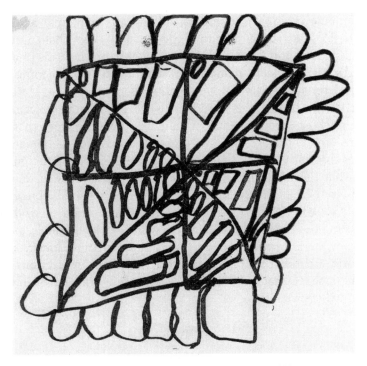

FIGURE 4.8. Mandala drawing by a 4-year-old boy.

as intrapsychic means of preventing outbursts and behavioral disinte-
gration" (p. 6).

In my own practice with children of this age, I have rarely seen
the diagrammatic and design-like forms that Rhoda Kellogg notes in
her work. At one point early in my career as an art therapist I became
intrigued with the fact that I did not observe what Kellogg had described and observed the drawings and art-making activity of approximately 100 children between from the ages of 3 to 4 years in a
preschool setting. At that time, I saw only two children who made
what might be called diagrams, combinations of forms, or mandalas as
defined by Kellogg. For the most part, art expression included both
scribbles and representational forms, moving directly from disordered
scribbling to longitudinal and circular scribbling to forms such as rudimentary people. Mandalas in the form of well-developed circular
scribbles are plentiful (such as Figure 4.9), as are images that are reminiscent of handwriting and printing alphabets (Figure 4.10), but ones

that combine various shapes are possibly not as common as reported. How Kellogg arrived at her findings has also been challenged by Golomb (1990) and Gardner (1980). Golomb, on the basis of a formalized study, concluded that only 4% of children drew the forms that Kellogg described.

It is hard to say when children first begin to draw objects and people they see around them, but many researchers believe that this happens around the age of 3 or 4 years. Rhoda Kellogg, for example, believes that early shapes and designs children draw are not connected to what they see. Others think that children are always drawing what is in their environment, and these perceptions are represented through scribbles and other early mark-making. There is evidence that during the time children begin to name or label scribbles or designs they are also making connections between their drawings and the world around them. They may begin to point to sections of a scribble or shape that remind them of something they have seen (an

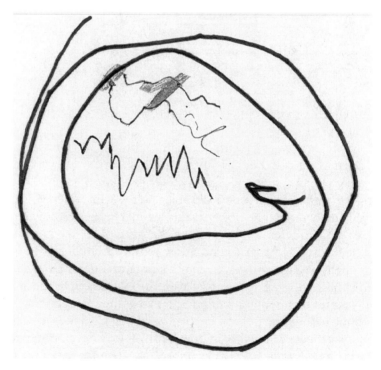

FIGURE 4.9. Mandala drawing by a 4-year-old girl.

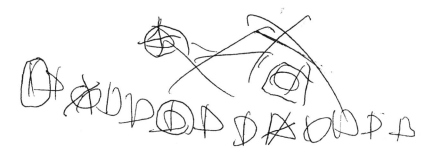

FIGURE 4.10. Drawing reminiscent of handwriting by a 3-year-old boy.

apple, a bird) after the drawing has been completed. Children at about this age often find abstract paintings more preferable than realistic ones according to Gardner (1982) because of their colors and design, and they are more able to identify a specific image in them such as a toy or other object. It is clear that imaginative thinking is a major developmental milestone for this stage in artistic development.

Stage III: Human Forms and Beginning Schemata

This stage is also part of the preoperational period (ages 4 to 7 years), particularly the latter part that includes increased symbolic thought, the ability to classify and see relationships, and the ability to understand numbers (Piaget, 1959). Of particular importance during this time are the children's spatial concepts, and they generally conceive space as being primarily related to themselves and their own bodies. In fact, a child's conception of the environment may be so strongly connected to him- or herself that his or her thoughts and feelings are confused with people or things around the child. For example, if a lamp falls and breaks, the child may be concerned with the lamp's being "hurt," as if the child were the lamp.

As previously noted, the most important development in this stage is the emergence of rudimentary human figures, often called tadpoles, because they resemble the first stage of a frog (Lowenfeld & Brittain, 1982) (Figure 4.11). These human figures are often primitive and sometimes quite charming. Although there may be some slight graphic differences in a particular child's tadpole drawings, they often appear the same even though each may represent different people

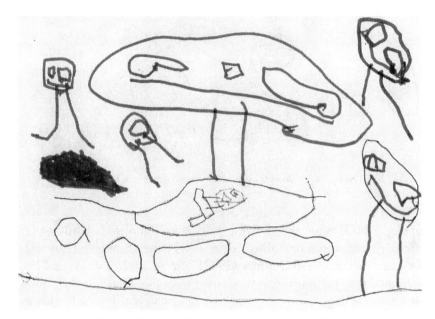

FIGURE 4.11. Tadpole drawings by a 4-year-old boy.

(e.g. mother, father, sister, baby). These first human figure drawings generally surface in children's art expressions anywhere from the ages of 4 to 6 years, although for some children, they occur even earlier. There may be a few false starts, however, and some children may revert back to scribbling for a few months before drawing another person.

Tadpole figures are thought to consist of a rudimentary head (a circle) and often two legs (two lines from the circle) and less frequently arms (two lines on either side of the circle). The head sometimes has facial features (eyes, nose, and mouth) and once in a while, a belly button in the center. For this reason, it has been argued by some that the circular portion thought to be a head is also representative of both head and trunk (Arnheim, 1974). Arnheim (1974) notes that children may try to create the simplest form that can be recognized as human, and since they have a limited graphic vocabulary, they reduce figures to simple geometric shapes. Cox and Parkin (1986) noted a transitional tadpole figure in which some children draw a circular head, with features such as arms, belly buttons, or buttons on clothing drawn below the head. Not all children draw this transitional figure, apparently for most, the head describes both the head and body of the

figure during this stage. When asked, children may say that their tadpole has no body because they cannot draw one or, on the other hand,
they may show you exactly where it is on the figure. Most children
seem to see it as part of the head and a smaller portion state that it is
located between the legs (Cox, 1989).

There is still a subjective use of color at this stage, although some
children may begin to associate color in their drawings with what they
perceive to be in the environment (e.g., leaves are green). Children of
this age are more interested in drawing the figure or object than the
color of it. Because color is still chosen subjectively, it is difficult to
determine if unusual use of color is anything other than the normal
experimentation with materials that occurs at this time. In the normal
child, drawings are free and often whimsical and inventive; there are
no rules, and the sun may be purple and the cow yellow.

Lowenfeld (1947; Lowenfeld & Brittain, 1982) refers to this time
as the preschematic stage of artistic development, emphasizing the
discovery of relationships among drawing, thinking, and reality. Also,
there is no conscious approach to composition or design, and children
may place objects throughout a page without concern for a groundline
or relationships to size (Figure 4.12). A figure may float freely across
the page, at the top or sides, and some things may be appear upside
down since children are not concerned with direction or relationship
of objects. This lack of concern for spatial placement coincides with
preoperational thinking, a period where when spatial relationships
have yet to be established outside of children's concepts of themselves. However, while there may appear to be no logic to the placement of objects on a page, the child may have a personal visual logic
(Winner, 1982) that rules his or her layout of forms; this is considered
to be a normal aspect of developing artistic expression.

Since human figures, often in the form of self-portraits or of family members, are popular themes, therapists, school counselors, and
psychologists who routinely look at human figure drawings for details
and omissions should be aware that children may actually know more
than they include in their tadpole drawings. Golomb (1990) found
that children know more about the human figure than they draw. She
discovered that when young children were asked to name various
body parts, they usually mentioned arms but often omitted them from
their human figure drawings. She also found that if children were
asked to draw a person doing an activity that required arms (such as a
person throwing a ball), they were more likely to include them.

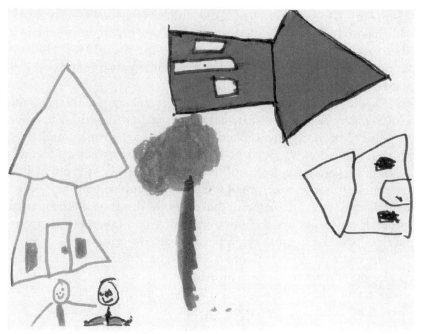

FIGURE 4.12. Drawing of houses without concern for groundline by a 5-year-old girl.

This underscores the importance of giving young children the opportunity to discuss their human figure drawings because they will often point out details that are not apparent to adult eyes. For example, a 4-year-old may draw a rudimentary human figure, but can describe in detail various parts of the body that are not obvious in the drawing, such as hands and fingers, lips, feet, and stomach. These simple figures stand for human beings and, to a child, describe the human body in greater detail than one would imagine.

Gradually, children become able to draw figures that are more differentiated from one another. The single circle initially used to denote both head and trunk may become two circles, or a circle and another form that stands for the trunk. Toward the end of this stage, most children will begin to include more features and characteristics such as toes and fingers, teeth, eyebrows, hair, and ears (Figure 4.13). Individuals of different sizes and shapes appear, and there is a slightly different representation for a baby, a father, a sister, and sometimes characters that are on television or read about in books. There are also rudimentary animals, at first looking like tadpoles with more legs (i.e.,

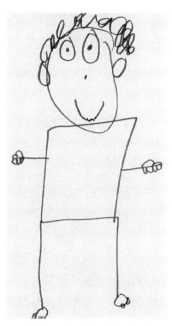

FIGURE 4.13. A 5½-year-old girl's drawing of a person including toes, fingers, hair, and ears.

a dog or a horse). Children also develop a schema for houses from rectilinear shapes, and their first identifiable images of common things in the environment such as the sun, flowers, and trees. In later years (as in the next three stages), children become more attracted to realism and leave simplicity to go on to more complex characteristics in their art expressions.

Stage IV: Development of a Visual Schema

Stage IV, the development of a visual schema for art expression, reflects the child's cognitive abilities at the latter part of the preoperational period and the beginning of concrete operations. Children are able to understand concepts of conservation and weight, they can arrange items in a series, and are beginning to be able to organize conceptually (Piaget, 1959; Piaget & Inhelder, 1971). They also become less egocentric and are able to represent objects in relation to one another rather than only in relation to themselves. During this developmental period, according to Piaget (1959), children seek to find order in the environment and to develop rules for behavior and structure in their lives (e.g., avoid stepping on cracks in the sidewalk and other personal rituals). This development of a schema for behavior is also apparent in how children express themselves through drawing and other creative expression.

From the ages of 6 to 9 years, children rapidly progress in their artistic abilities. The first and foremost of these abilities is the development of visual symbols or true schemata (Lowenfeld, 1947; Lowenfeld & Brittain, 1982) for human figures, animals, houses, trees, and other objects in the environment. Many of these symbols are fairly standard to most children's drawings, such as a particular way to depict a person with a circular head, hairstyle, arms, and legs; a tree often with a brown trunk and green top; a yellow sun in the corner of the page; and a house with a triangular, pitched roof (Figure 4.14). There is a discovery of relationship between color and objects,and sometimes color is even used rigidly (e.g., all leaves must be the same color green).

The tadpole of the previous stage is fully replaced by a human

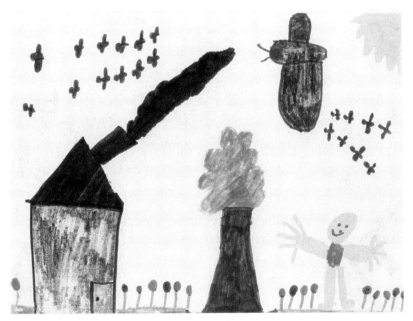

FIGURE 4.14. Schematic drawing of a person, house, tree, flowers, and bees by a 6½-year-old boy.

figure with a head and a trunk, as well as additional details, and the figure now usually sits on a baseline, either drawn at the bottom of the paper or implied by the paper's edge. In addition to this groundline upon which objects sit, there may also be a skyline (a line across the top the drawing, often blue, to indicate the sky). While children may include groundlines or skylines, there is no attempt yet to represent the world in a truly three-dimensional way.

At 6 years, an average child is unable to represent depth. For example, when drawing a table, a simple profile view may be used and the objects that are on that table are sometimes drawn as floating above it. By ages 7 or 8 the table is still drawn in the same way, but objects now sit on the top of the table. They also may try to show three dimensions by drawing a bird's eye view of a table top, in addition to including all four legs of the table extended outward from the surface (Figure 4.15). This phenomenon is referred to as "folding-over" (Lowenfeld, 1942; Lowenfeld & Brittain, 1982). Children may also draw a car showing all four wheels or a chair with all four legs. By the end of this stage, some children may draw two separate groundlines,

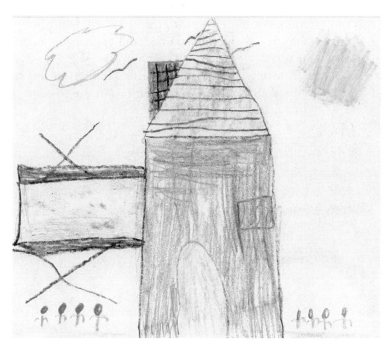

FIGURE 4.15. A 7-year-old girl's drawing of a picnic table illustrating "folding-over."

indicating one of the first true attempts at depth in their images (Figure 4.16) and also may include a rudimentary form of perspective by placing more distant objects higher on the drawing page.

Children also draw see-through or X-ray pictures (Figure 4.17, showing a cut-away image of a house) where one can see everything inside. Winner (1982) notes that there are actually two different types of X-ray drawings. One includes drawings that show the contents of the inside of an object or thing, such as depicting what is in an animal's stomach. The other type of X-ray drawing involves transparency—in order to show that a person is behind a table. For example, the child may draw a transparent table allowing the figure to show through from behind.

Drawings made by children in Stage III and the early part of Stage IV are often thought to be quite charming, free of rules or conventions, and often, to the adult eye, beautifully colored. Researchers who have studied extensively children's artistic development frequently note that art expressions from this age range are very creative and uninhibited, representing the "golden age of artistic expression" (Gardner, 1980) and resemble in some ways the work of modern artists (Winner, 1982). Whether or not the drawings of children during this time are more or less esthetic to the eye is still being debated; what is undeniably true is the unrestrained and enchanting qualities of many of the images.

Exaggerations in size are one element that children in this stage use freely. It is normal at this age to use variations in size to emphasize

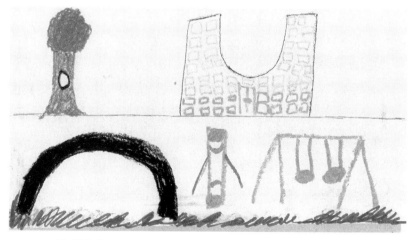

FIGURE 4.16. Drawing with two groundlines by a 9-year-old girl.

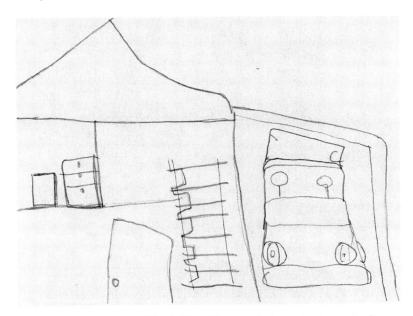

FIGURE 4.17. A 9-year-old boy's "X-ray" drawing of a house showing car in the garage and stairs and dresser in the house.

importance; for example, the child may depict him- or herself as bigger than the house or tree in the same drawing, if she or he wishes to emphasize the figure. Or a child depicting a person throwing a ball may draw a much longer arm than usual. Joey, a 7-year-old boy wanted to show me how happy he was about his family moving to a brand new house and drew himself with an emphasized, wide-mouthed, and toothy grin (Figure 4.18). Another boy proudly drew himself with a large felt marker in hand because, as he told me, "I am drawing with a green marker!" (Figure 4.19). Also, unimportant details may be eliminated; for example, if a child is drawing a person throwing a ball, he or she may leave off a body part that is unimportant to the picture (e.g., ears on a face).

These exaggerations or emphasized elements or omissions in images are important when looking at children's drawings for unusual characteristics, for at this particular developmental stage, it is difficult to say if enlargements, dramatic emphases, or even obvious omissions of details are unusual and of concern. In many cases, these characteristics are part of the normal developmental process of a particular child. For example, Joey's toothy grin might be interpreted as hostility by

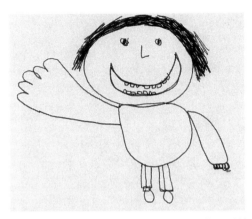

FIGURE 4.18. Seven-year-old Joey's drawing of himself smiling.

some (especially if one is considering his drawing from characteristics listed in some projective drawing tests), since teeth are considered by some to be indications of aggressiveness, rather than pure joy he was expressing in this situation. Although Joey's self-portrait could be understood in a variety of ways and from different perspectives, it does demonstrate the aspect of exaggeration that is common at this stage from developmental viewpoint and meaningful within that context.

There are circumstances in which children use exaggeration of an element, form, or object both because the child wants to emphasize

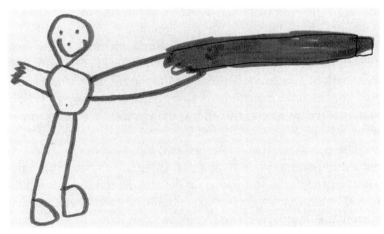

FIGURE 4.19. "I am drawing with a green marker!" A 6-year-old boy's drawing of himself with a large green felt marker.

something to the viewer and also as a result of some experience of trauma. Figure 4.14, previously shown as an example of typical drawing style of this stage, demonstrates this. The child who drew this picture was recently stung by a bee and was understandably quite traumatized by the experience. The "bad" bee that stung the child is shown as the largest figure in the upper half of the drawing, flying overhead with other smaller bees, and emphasized through its size when compared to the others. (There is also a theme of repetition, i.e., many repeated images of bees, something that may be characteristic of traumatized children's drawings, a topic that is discussed in more detail in Chapter 5.)

Finally, there is an increasing ability to create time sequences (e.g., images showing travel, journeys, a batter hitting a ball), drawings that imply that a series of events will happen. For example, 6-year-old Ian's drawing of a baseball pitcher who has just pitched the ball to the batter now watches the ball flying overhead (Figure 4.20). This simple drawing implies many things—that the pitcher has thrown the ball, the batter has hit it, and it is now going out of the ballpark (according to Ian's description of the outcome). These aspects of storyline and time sequences, along with the emergence of X-ray pictures, are two developmental themes that therapists or teachers working with children may want to use to stimulate drawing in children in this age range.

Stage V: Realism

During this stage of artistic development (about ages 9 through 12), the period of concrete operations continues, and children continue to shift away from egocentric thinking. Children begin to consider the thoughts, opinions, and feelings of others. Their understanding of interrelationships, cause and effect, and interdependence is just starting, laying the groundwork for the ability to work within groups. Children of this age also become increasingly aware of the world around them, and earlier modes of expression (i.e., schematic representations) no longer satisfy children's needs to represent their perceptions in their drawings.

Generally, by the age of 9 or 10, children become very interested in depicting what they perceive to be realistic elements in their drawings. There is a movement away from schematic representations and

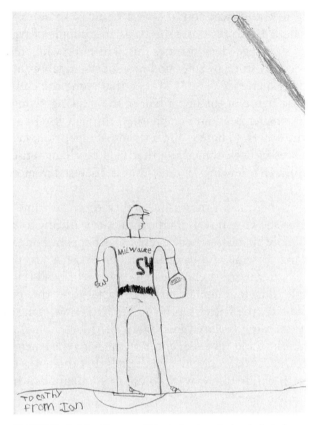

FIGURE 4.20. Six-year-old Ian's drawing of a baseball pitcher.

increasing complexity in what is represented through line, shape, and detail. This includes the first attempts at perspective. Children no longer draw a simple baseline, but, instead, draw the ground meeting the sky to create depth. There is a more accurate depiction of color in nature (e.g., leaves can be many different colors, rather than just one shade of green), and the human figure is more detailed and differentiated in gender characteristics (e.g., more details in hair, clothing, and build) (Figure 4.21).

Many researchers who have studied children's art believe that drawings done at this age are much less free and less charming than ones done at earlier stages. In reality, children now begin to become more conventional in their art expressions and are more literal because they want to achieve a more "photographic effect" to their renditions. Children in Stage V are less able to conjure up imaginary

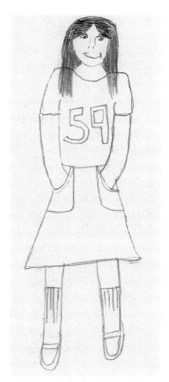

FIGURE 4.21. Drawing of a human figure by an 11-year-old girl.

worlds than when they were at 4 or 5 years. Everything is seen from a literal viewpoint, and children believe that the more accurately one can depict an object, person, or environment, the better the art expression. The beginning of this interest in realism starts, however, in the previous stage. Around the age of 6 or 7 years, children's interest in the real world begins to dominate, and they begin to prefer traditional paintings that are more realistic and even may state that photographs are better than painting since they are more lifelike (Gardner, 1982).

Children also realize that the fold-over qualities in earlier attempts at perspective are incorrect and work to correctly approximate the third dimension. For example, children may now be able to draw a table top as a rectangle with two legs in front and two smaller legs behind. A study by Willats (1977) examined the progressive changes in how children from 5 to 17 years draw objects as they saw them on a table (Figure 4.22). Willats' study found that the youngest children

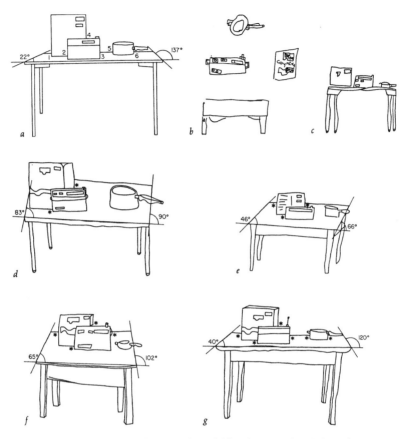

FIGURE 4.22. Progressive changes in how children from ages 5 to 17 draw objects seen on a table. (a) Correct perspective drawing of table, showing angle size and six points of overlap. (b) Stage I drawing, with no depth or overlap and objects floating above the table top. (c) Stage II drawing, with no depth or overlap; table top shown from the side so that only the edge is visible. (d) Stage III drawing, with back–front relations represented by top–bottom relations (asterisks indicate overlap). (e) Stage IV drawing, with table top drawn as a parallelogram. (f) Stage V drawing, with naive perspective, lines converging only slightly. (g) Stage VI drawing, with correct perspective, lines converging according to the laws of optics. From "How Children Learn to Draw Realistic Pictures" by J. Willats, in *Quarterly Journal of Experimental Psychology, 29,* 367–382. Copyright 1977 by The Experimental Psychology Society. Reprinted by permission.

drew a rectangle to represent the table and drew the objects floating above it. By ages 7 or 8, children drew a straight line for the table and placed the objects on that line; the line seemed to serve a similar function to that of the schematic baseline previously described in Stage IV. At age 9, children began to graphically represent depth, drawing a table top with parallel sides, and including the objects on the table's surface. Following this, children gradually began to draw a more accurate parallelogram for the table top but lack true perspective. Finally, adolescents (Stage VI) were able to draw in perspective: The far side of the table was drawn smaller than the near side.

It is important to remember that children at this stage are so concerned with perfection of their drawings that they may compose and develop drawings in ways much different from earlier years. For example, there is less of a concern with composition and children are more interested in how things look rather than where they are on the page. Children may also leave out features that they feel that they cannot perfect or draw well—for example, drawing hands held behind the body because they are hard to draw in a realistically satisfying way.

It is not surprising that cartoon images or caricatures become popular at this stage. When asked to make a drawing of a person, children and preadolescents may now prefer to make drawings of cartoon or comic-strip characters in order to feel comfortable with the quality of their pictures. Because the features of cartoon characters can be exaggerated, absurd, or outrageous, they allow for some lack of technical competence or photographic correctness required to draw human figures (Figure 4.23). However, some children at this stage resort to stereotype images (rather than creating unique images of their own) or prefer to copy.

During this stage, many children become discouraged and may

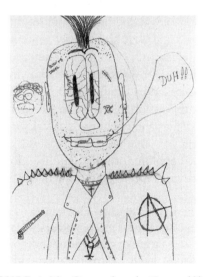

FIGURE 4.23. Cartoon figure by 12-year-old boy.

not draw again, except if they are encouraged by parents or take art courses in middle or high school. For this reason, many drawings done by adults (including those of you reading this book) look like children's drawings at the age of 10 or 11. People continue to progress in other areas of development, such as language, but the development of drawing skills may not persist. Indeed, Lindstrom (1957) noted:

> Discontented with his own accomplishments and extremely anxious to please others with his art, he tends to give up original creation and personal expression . . . further development of his visualizing powers and even his capacity for original thought and for relating himself through personal feelings to his environment may be blocked at this point. It is a crucial stage beyond which many adults have not advanced. (p. 13)

This is important for therapists to know not only in their work with children but also with adults who make drawings or other art expressions as part of their therapy. Over many years of work with adults, I have often heard them relate their painful memories of not being able to draw or feel comfortable with expressing themselves through art. They also may relate frustrations with the process of drawing (e.g., "I can't make it look real" or "I am not talented in art"), just as children in this stage speak of their frustrations with perfecting the realism of their drawings. Others may remember someone's uncomplimentary remarks about the drawings they made as children, perhaps a thoughtless comment from a teacher, family member, or friend. My colleague Ewa, who holds a doctoral degree in anthropology and two master's degrees, told me that she clearly remembers when she was about 9 or 10 her elementary school teacher proclaiming, "What a nice sewing machine" upon looking at her drawing of a horse. Obviously, she was discouraged by the teacher's comments, and it probably was a particularly impressionable time in her drawing development, reinforcing the idea that she could not draw. Ewa never felt comfortable with art again.

Gardner (1980) explores other possibilities for why children may move away from previous interests in drawing.

> There is yet another possibility—children may simply conclude that their feelings can no longer be captured graphically or that drawing is no longer a suitable means of confronting one's own feeling . . . expressive drawing is most likely to involve those children whose developmental course has been unusually rocky—those who, owing to personal

or family problems, intellectual or social difficulties, have not yet suc-
cumbed to the pressures molding other youngsters. (p. 152)

However, Gardner concludes that neither of these ideas is truly plausi-
ble. What may be most likely is that there are now a number of other
ways to express oneself, particularly language, which is encouraged in
schools and is useful in communicating with peers who become important during this time. For whatever reason, drawing development
has usually halted for most individuals by the end of this stage, either
due to lack of exposure or encouragement to draw, or to negative feedback or self-criticism.

Stage VI: Adolescence

The stage of adolescence, although not the primary subject of this
book, is nonetheless important to understanding the full range of children's drawing development. As already mentioned, many adults never reach this stage of artistic development because they may discon-
tinue drawing or making art at around the age of 10 or 11 due to other
interests or feelings of discouragement over lack of technical competence. Therefore, in working with teenagers, one should realize that
many of them may have stopped developing in their artistic skills and
experience with drawing. It therefore may be quite normal to see adolescents draw in Stage V style, particularly if they have little or no additional exposure to art making past that time. Therapists may also
find some normal resistance to drawing for some of the reasons described in the previous section.

However, by the age of 13 or 14 years, children who have continued to make art will be able to use perspective more accurately and effectively in their drawings; will include greater detail in their work;
will have an increasing critical perception of the environment; will
have increasing mastery of materials; will be more attentive to color
and design; and will be able to create abstract images. When young
people are encouraged and given the opportunity to continue to develop and improve skills in drawing, their work can be quite impressive, detailed, thoughtful, and creative in both style and content (Figures 4.24 and 4.25).

Some adolescents progress to artistic skills of adult artists not
only because they have sophisticated technical competencies but also

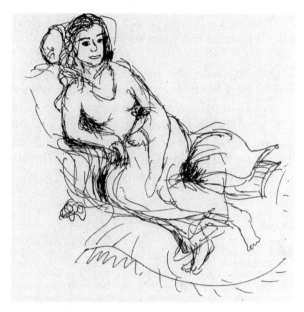

FIGURE 4.24. A 16-year-old girl's self-portrait.

because they begin to make choices about how they portray an object, person, or scene. For example, in creating a still life, the adolescent who drew it thought carefully about how to render the images to create a mood and personal statement (Figure 4.25). While younger children focus on making images of people, animals, and environments, adolescents may use those elements not only as part of their compositions but also to purposefully symbolize and communicate ideas about issues, personal philosophies, and themselves.

THE IMPORTANCE OF DEVELOPMENTAL ASPECTS OF CHILDREN'S DRAWINGS

The developmental stages of children's artistic expression are a foundation for understanding children's drawings in general. Knowing what is "normal" or expected for a particular age group provides a baseline for comparing what is unusual or unexpected in children's drawings. Understanding children's drawings through a developmental lens not only provides information important to evaluation, but it also establishes a starting point for creating effective interventions.

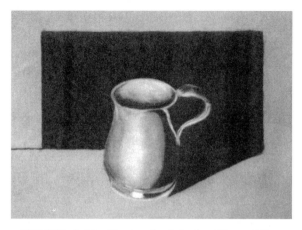

FIGURE 4.25. Drawing of a pitcher by a 17-year-old boy.

Although knowing and recognizing developmental characteristics in children's drawings is important to any work with children's art expressions, there are circumstances when it may be not only useful but essential. Developmental characteristics are particularly helpful in work with children who have developmental delays, learning disabilities, or some form of mental retardation. In general, children with learning disabilities or mental retardation may show some developmental delays in their art expression, depending on the type of disability and other factors. For example, both a learning-disabled 7-year-old and a mentally retarded adolescent may still be engaged in scribbling, finding success in holding a crayon or felt pen, and making somewhat controlled scribbles on paper. In the latter case, scribbled lines and random marks on paper may characterize children's art expressions for many years beyond the expected ages for scribbling.

Learning disabilities include perceptual and neurological impairments, specific learning problems (such as reading comprehension), attention-deficit disorders, and dyslexia, and therefore, the characteristics and developmental aspects of drawings made by children with learning disabilities can be quite variable. There is no set way that learning disabilities present themselves through children's art expressions; in fact, the drawings of children with learning disabilities may be affected by many factors in addition to development. However, art expression can provide a great deal of information pertinent to the development of cognitive and perceptual skills.

Children with developmental disabilities may be restricted in their use of themes, produce stereotypical images, or be limited in their abilities to experiment with materials. A therapist or teacher who works with children with significant developmental problems may not see much progression to other stages even over long periods of time; or, when changes do occur, they may appear in small increments. Art activities, such as drawing, may be more in the area of exploratory activities. Although the creation of a symbolic image with personal meaning may be a therapeutic goal, content may not be as much of an issue as experimentation with materials for many of these children.

In working with children through their drawings, it is helpful to think about some questions concerning development. One area that might be considered is the type of media used to make drawings. Could adaptations be helpful to the child in terms of self-expression? For example, would larger pencils that make broad lines be helpful or smaller drawing instruments that allow for more articulation of line? Does the child have an aversion to some materials (such as "messy" materials like chalk)? Adaptations in materials and drawing surface may have an effect on the developmentally delayed child's experience with drawing.

DRAWINGS AS MEASURES OF CREATIVE AND COGNITIVE CAPACITIES

Although learning disabilities, retardation, and other impairments may affect the content and quality of art expression, some developmental aspects have been more closely examined using drawings as measures of creative and cognitive abilities. As mentioned in Chapter 1, drawings have been used as measures of intelligence and cognition (Harris, 1963; Koppitz, 1968). This use of standardized drawing tests, usually involving a human figure drawing, has relied on developmental aspects of children's art expressions, but it has been limited in scope when considering the complexities of composition, spatial relationships, and mental operations that go into drawing. As described in this chapter, children's drawings involve far more than just inclusion of details or omissions; aspects such as the ability to combine line and shape, to relate objects to each other on paper, and to create depth and perspective are a few of the many components that must be considered when looking at children's art expressions.

Silver (1978, 1992, 1993, 1996) has devoted many years of research to understanding both creative and cognitive aspects of children from a developmental perspective. The Silver Drawing Test (SDT) is one part of Silver's work in this area and was initially developed when she considered the links between art expression and intelligence. The SDT evolved from Silver's hypothesis that the intelligence of children who have poor language skills is often underestimated. She saw the possibilities that art expression could have in understanding children's abilities and noted that, through drawing and other art activities, children with poor language skills (or those who have difficulty understanding others or making themselves understood) might be able to express themselves more easily than through words.

Silver devised a series of drawing tasks that assess a child's ability to solve conceptual problems in a graphic manner. She focused on three areas as measures of cognitive development: predictive or sequential drawing, drawing from observation, and drawing from the imagination. While drawing tests such as the Draw-A-Person are limited to drawing specific items, Silver's activities are more broad in scope, involving a series of interesting tasks and allowing the child to choose and adapt images in drawing. The drawing activities involve both structured protocols (a predictive drawing task and a drawing from observation of a simple still life) as well as less structured opportunities to draw from imagination through choosing from a series of images and combining them in a drawing and providing a title and story.

In relation to developmental milestones, Silver's predictive drawing tasks and the task designed to allow children to draw from observation are the most pertinent to this chapter. The purpose of the predictive drawing task is to measure how well children can deal with concepts of horizontality, verticality, and sequencing. Children are first asked to use their predictive skills by adding lines to empty soda glasses to show the way the soda would look if emptied gradually (Figure 4.26) and to show the way water would look if a bottle were tilted in a certain way. The third task involves drawing a house on a steep slope. Silver has devised a scale to score these three areas of predictability, the higher scores on a 5-point scale indicating more advanced skills.

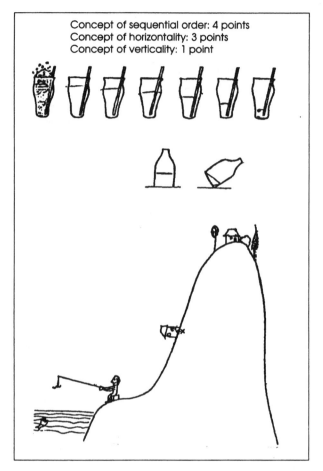

FIGURE 4.26. Silver's test of predictive skills. From *Silver Drawing Test of Cognition and Emotion* (3rd ed.) by Rawley Silver. Copyright 1996 by Rawley Silver. Reprinted by permission.

These three tasks are significant in terms of understanding children's stages of cognitive development. For example, the soda glass exercise has particular significance in understanding a child's developing ability to work with the idea of sequencing, a skill important to understanding cause and effect and conservation. The water bottle exercise underscores the concept of horizontality; for example, at 4 or 5 years, children tend to scribble round forms when asked to draw water in bottles. Gradually, they learn to draw lines parallel to the base of the bottle, even when the bottle is tilted. By about the age of 9 most children draw horizontal lines in the tilted bottle, demonstrating an understanding of horizontality.

The concept of verticality is evident in the drawing of the house on a hillside. According to Silver (1996a) children asked to draw houses on the side of a mountain will draw them inside the outline of the mountain. Later, children draw them perpendicular to the side of the mountain, and finally, by the age of 8 or 9, they are more likely to draw them upright.

The drawing activity involving observation emphasizes the ability to deal with spatial concepts. The test developed by Silver is similar to the study by Willats (1977) that had children from 5 to 17 years draw objects as they saw them on a table (Figure 4.27). Silver's exercise involves drawing an arrangement of three cylinders that differ in height and width and a small stone or object. Drawing the four items (the cylinders and the stone or object) helps to determine whether the child has acquired the ability to represent spatial relationships involving height, width, and depth.

Silver's work, although developed as a standardized test of cognition and emotion (her work on emotion is addressed in Chapter 5), is significant in that it provides important information for therapists, teachers, and others who work with children. How children conceptualize space and how they demonstrate conservation through sequencing, horizontality, and verticality are all evident in their drawings. A clear understanding of how these factors appear throughout early and late childhood is intrinsic to fully comprehending the content of children's drawings. A very brief overview of Silver's extensive

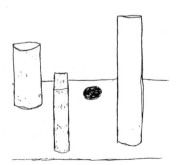

FIGURE 4.27. Silver's test for ability to deal with spatial concepts: Drawing objects on a table. From *Silver Drawing Test of Cognition and Emotion* (3rd ed.) by Rawley Silver. Copyright 1996 by Rawley Silver. Reprinted by permission.

work in this area has been provided here, and readers are referred to her most recent text, *Silver Drawing Test of Cognition and Emotion* (1996a), for more in-depth information.

UNUSUAL DRAWING ABILITIES

There are times when a therapist may see a child with what appears to be unusual or gifted drawing abilities. Therapists may be impressed with many children's drawings, thinking that the children's drawing abilities even surpass their own. Since the average adult, for the most part, draws like a 10-year-old, it is easy to understand how many therapists would be impressed with some children's more advanced artistic talents. However, skills in copying or creating photographic likenesses can easily be mistaken for unusual or true giftedness in the area of drawing or art expression. In reality, there are relatively few children whose drawing abilities would be considered "gifted," although their abilities and proficiencies are impressive.

There are a few reported cases of unusual drawing abilities in children that have captured the interest of researchers, particularly those interested in human development and creative expression. The extraordinary case of Nadia, a young girl diagnosed as functionally retarded with autistic affect, is one of few examples. Nadia has been the subject of an in-depth study (Selfe, 1977) and has been explored by many others in both the fields of art and psychology (Gardner, 1979; Winner, 1986; Henley, 1989, 1992). Despite profound handicaps and lacking functional language, Nadia, from ages 3 years to 6 years, created drawings that rivaled those of adult artists (see Figures 4.28 and 4.29). Her giftedness emerged spontaneously and defied the principles of developmental stages in artistic expression. However, this extraordinary ability lasted only a few years, and by the time Nadia was a young adult, her work had deteriorated to that characteristic of a person with severe mental retardation (see Figure 4.30). This disappearance of her artistic proclivity into a regressive style of expression makes her case both unusual and mysterious.

Although it is highly unlikely that most therapists or teachers will work with a child of Nadia's extraordinary abilities, her case brings to light the many questions that still are unanswered about artistic development in children. Certainly, the relationship between artistic talent and measurable intelligence comes into question. Hen-

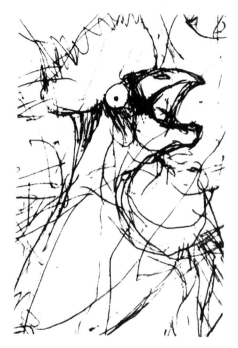

FIGURE 4.28. Drawing by Nadia as a young child. From *Nadia: A Case of Extraordinary Drawing Ability in an Austic Child* by Lorna Selfe. Copyright 1977 by the Academic Press Limited London. Reprinted by permission. Photo by David Henley.

ley (1989, 1992), in his work with Nadia as a young adult, notes that her interest in drawing, the outpouring of drawings at certain times, the changes in her work, and apparent deterioration in her drawing abilities may be related to her crises with separation from and eventual loss of her mother. About Nadia and her remarkable drawings, Henley (1989) observes:

> Despite Nadia's blazing artistic output, she failed to thrive. Neither self-help nor academic skills advanced although she received a great deal of speech therapy and other special education. Nadia's expressive language never attained a fully functioning status and her behavior remained autistic. Her emotional development suffered further setbacks as the mother, suffering from cancer eventually died; at this time, the child began to phase out drawing altogether. (p. 46)

Although Nadia's deterioration in artistic expression has been connected to cognitive, language, and neurological deficits, Henley's

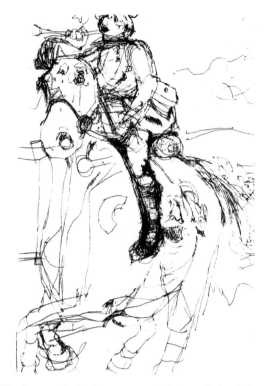

FIGURE 4.29. Drawing by Nadia as young child. From *Nadia: A Case of Extraordinary Drawing Ability in an Austic Child* by Lorna Selfe. Copyright 1977 by the Academic Press Limited London. Reprinted by permission. Photo by David Henley.

work with Nadia led him to explore the connections between the child's drawings and emotional trauma. He observed that Nadia began drawing at the time of her mother's discharge from a lengthy hospital stay; she also may have used drawing at other times to adapt and cope with her feelings in response to her feelings of abandonment when separated from her mother. Henley's conclusions (1989) bring up interesting questions about the connections between developmental aspects of art expression and emotion, the subject of Chapter 5.

CONCLUSION

The developmental stages of children artistic expression form a rich foundation for understanding children's drawings in general. The fact

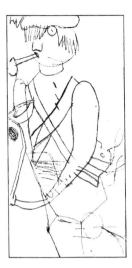

FIGURE 4.30. Drawing by Nadia as a young adult. From *Nadia: A Case of Extraordinary Drawing Ability in an Austic Child* by Lorna Selfe. Copyright 1977 by the Academic Press Limited London. Reprinted by permission. Photo by David Henley.

that most children follow a fairly predictable sequence is a good starting point for therapists in their evaluation of children's drawings. The stages presented in this chapter can be used as the basis for assessment of children's drawings, providing therapists with a framework for thinking about children's expressive work through a developmental lens that can help to identify and distinguish delays in cognitive and perceptual growth.

Although there is an extensive amount of research on developmental aspects of children's art expressions, there are still many unanswered questions. For example, children may progress to another stage of development and, just as suddenly, regress to an earlier form of artistic behavior. Exactly why many children move back and forth between stages described by Lowenfeld (1947, 1982), Gardner (1979, 1980), and others is not always obvious. How external influences such as parents, teachers, and peers, or society and culture impact artistic development is another area that is still not well-defined. Also, how gender may affect children's drawings at various developmental levels is still not completely understood (see Chapter 6 for a discussion of gender and children's art expressions), remaining a perplexing question of nature (i.e., biological inheritance) versus nurture (i.e., influence of society).

What is important to remember with regard to development and drawing is that children's artistic development is not a strictly vertical process and that many factors in children's lives will influence this development. Because artistic development is shaped by many factors, including emotional, cognitive, social, and physical growth, progression and regression in drawing style may be the result of one or many of these influences. Children who are under a great of emotional stress because of trauma, loss, or crisis in their lives will often show fluctuations in developmental aspects of their drawings. As described in Chapter 5, developmental aspects are salient to the therapist's understanding of the content and style of children's art expressions, providing some important information on children's abilities to deal with stressful situations or emotional disturbances.

Lastly, as Lowenfeld and Brittain (1982) noted, "Drawing gives us a good indication of the child's growth, moving from an egocentric point of view to gradual awareness of the self as part of a larger environment" (p. 52) and emphasized that art expression is reflective of "total" growth in children. In this sense, the developmental aspects of children's art have the possibility to relate more than just cognitive improvement and intellectual progress. Drawings are reflective of not only the children themselves but also of their emerging development with regard to interpersonal development—that is, how children see, perceive, and respond to the world around them, the subject of Chapter 6. Children's drawings provide a unique frame of reference for thinking about and evaluating children's overall development in many areas, and, for this reason, they offer therapists a unique way of understanding children from a variety of developmental perspectives.

Emotional Content
of Children's Drawings

Arnheim (1992) observed that art serves as

> a helper in times of trouble, as a means of understanding the conditions of human existence and of facing the frightening aspects of those conditions, [and] as the creation of a meaningful order offering a refuge from the unmanageable confusion of the outer reality. (p. 170)

Most therapists who use drawings with children realize that art expression can be a powerful modality for those who are emotionally traumatized, disturbed, or grieving and is a way to contain and explore powerful and confusing feelings. For this reason, it is understandable that helping professionals are extremely interested in what art expressions can tell them about children's emotional lives. This is not surprising because art is a recognized way to communicate feelings and the majority of therapeutic interventions (including those involving art activities) with children often focus on the resolution of emotional crisis, trauma, or disturbance.

USES OF DRAWING IN DIAGNOSIS
AND TREATMENT

The use of art to interpret emotions began early in this century when interest grew in patients' drawings as aids in diagnosis of psychopathology and in understanding the psychological states of these individuals. However, in spite of the continuing interest in using art expressions to understand emotion, using art expressions to diagnose emotional or mental illness has been criticized, and some even feel that it is not possible to utilize drawings in this way (Golomb, 1990).

Despite this sentiment, children's art expressions continue to be explored for their diagnostic value. In particular, significant emphasis has been placed on understanding the content of drawings created by children who have been traumatized by physical or sexual abuse, violence, or other serious crises, possibly because children who have experienced severe trauma are often hesitant to talk about their feelings. Although most therapists would agree that children's art expressions are an important source of information about personality and emotions, there is relatively little reliable information to support specific interpretations of affective material in children's drawings. At best, there may be a few characteristics that consistently indicate emotional problems. Projective drawing tests have supported the idea that certain structural elements and symbols in drawings are indicative of emotional distress. However, as previously mentioned, evaluating children's work through single elements is problematic and often counterproductive to fully understanding their experiences. There is also a great deal of clinical writing, particularly in the field of art therapy, acknowledging the connection between children's art expressions and their emotional experiences, but much of this material is based on case studies and opinions of clinical experts in the field rather than on quantifiable data. There has, however, been renewed exploration of children's drawings for possible diagnostic value in recent years (Neale, 1994; Sobol & Cox, 1992).

Notwithstanding controversy in using drawings in diagnosis, the field of art therapy continues to explore the ideas that children's art expressions are containers for feelings and that the expression of emotion through art has inherent therapeutic value. The fundamental tenets of art therapy involve communication, control, and resolution of emotional conflicts through art making (American Art Therapy Association, 1996). These concepts are closely related to psychodynamic theories that emphasize the connection between unresolved feelings and emotional adjustment. Experiences such as catharsis (the expression of suppressed feelings) are thought to be an important part of the art therapy process in that drawing or other forms of artistic activity may help children to resolve emotional problems and tensions through image making. For example, a child who draws an image of his anger at his sister may gain some relief from communicating conflictual feelings about the situation through art. Also, for children who lack the ability to communicate emotions verbally, art expression is believed to bring order and containment to feelings that may be contradictory, confusing, or difficult to say with words.

Kramer (1993) underscored the healing potentials of the art process in terms of emotions, stressing that creativity, not merely the communication of visual symbols, is what is important. Of her work with child refugees from Nazi Germany, Kramer (1993) said:

> I first observed the different responses to stress as they manifested in children's art, responses that would later become very familiar to me. I saw regression; repetition that told of unresolved conflict; I first observed identification with the aggressor in children who identified with Hitler, who has proven his power by the very damage he had done to them; I saw withdrawal into frozen rigidity, and, finally, the capacity for creative expression surviving under difficulties. (p. xiv)

To deny that children express emotions through art would ignore a significant part of who they are and how they perceive themselves and the world around them. Art is a potent container for their emotional lives and is undeniably an important aspect of understanding children.

THE COMPLEXITIES OF EMOTIONAL CONTENT IN CHILDREN'S DRAWINGS

To begin to understand the emotional content of children's drawings, it is first important to respect their creative work for its complexities. Since emotional problems are not simple and are experienced differently by each child, looking at art to assess for emotional difficulties is not a simple task. Children's feelings are often complex, contradictory, and confusing to both the child and the adult who observes or works with the child. Fortunately, art is one of few modalities that can contain many emotions simultaneously.

Probably what is most difficult about understanding the emotional content of children's drawings is recognizing that our own emotions as adults get in the way. As previously mentioned, art evokes feeling from its viewers, and children's art expressions, particularly those created by children in emotional crisis, often evoke powerful feelings in those who witness them. Adults with an interest in children's art cannot help but project their own feelings of joy, anxiety, fear, or sadness into the color, lines, forms and content of children's work. Therapists can learn to recognize that they are affected by children's imagery in personal ways that may or may not be representative of what children are experiencing or conveying.

In early childhood art, it is difficult to say how children convey feelings through their drawings because the very idea of expressing emotion is an abstract concept for them. Very young children have a relatively limited visual vocabulary, and it is difficult at best to draw conclusions about their emotional states from their drawings. Children in the schematic stage (see Chapter 4), however, can depict more recognizable images of emotions. For example, when asked to make a picture of the feelings happy, angry, and sad, children will usually respond with images of a smiling face or a face with large teeth (happy), a frowning face or a crooked smile (angry), or tearful face (sad), or other frecognizable acial expressions in their drawings (Figure 5.1). Golomb (1990) notes that up until the age of 10, children use a face representationally to express emotion, using curved lines, eyebrows, and sometimes tears to express sadness when asked to express particular emotions. After the age of 10, bodies are more likely to be included, and features such as arms in different positions may be used to relate emotion.

To understand the symbolic content of children's spontaneous art expressions, structural elements, including line, shape, color, size, and overall organization, are equally important to observe. How these elements are expressed is influenced by the developmental characteristics discussed in Chapter 4. It is obvious that younger children generally have less motor control than older children, and this affects the quality of line, shape, and organization in their drawings. Again, it is important not to be overzealous in one's interpretation of structural elements. What may look like an anxious or distressed line to an adult eye can merely be a lack of ability to control materials or articulate with a pencil, marker, or crayon.

Color

How children use color to express emotion has received some emphasis over the years with respect to children's drawings. Since color is perceived to be closely related to feeling, it is difficult to look at it in

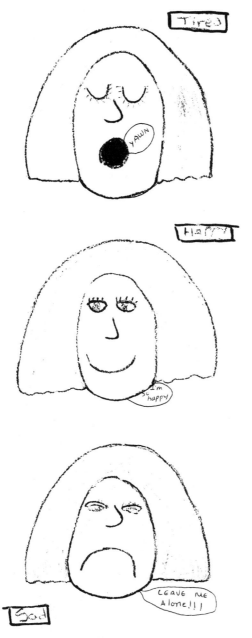

FIGURE 5.1. Drawing of emotions by a 9-year-old girl: tired, happy, and sad.

any art expression without reacting to it emotionally. Each individual brings notions about the meanings of color, many of which are connected to cultural and societal influences and traditions as well as personal meanings.

Because color has many emotional connotations, therapists naturally want to know if color has any particular meaning or diagnostic value especially with children who are emotionally troubled or traumatized. There is often concern about children who limit the use of color to one color in particular (i.e., monochromatic color usage), unusual uses of color, or emphasis of one color in a drawing over others. Although this may hold some meaning, it is important to remember that many factors govern how children use color in their art expressions.

When thinking about color in children's art, it is particularly important to recall the developmental norms for color usage at each stage. In the initial stages of artistic development (Stages I and II, from 18 months to 4 years), children are generally not conscious of color choices and will often grab whatever color crayon or marker is easiest to reach. Later (Stage III, ages 4 to 6 years), there is subjective use of color, although some children may begin to associate color in their drawings with what they perceive in the environment. This makes it difficult to determine if color has any particular meaning other than the usual experimentation with materials that occurs at this time. Golomb (1990) notes that children as young as four years start to use color representationally; although there is still considerable freedom in color choices, some uses are related to the object represented. In the next stage (Stage IV, ages 6 to 9 years), a schematic use of color emerges, and children develop rules for color in their drawings (e.g., a tree with a brown trunk and green top). Although color use can be more rigid and rule-oriented at this time, unusual use of color may be more easily noticed and have more significance than at previous stages. Older children (Stage V, ages 9 years and up) tend to use color realistically and are apt to use colors as they appear in nature in their drawings.

These are guidelines for children's use of color from a developmental model, and there may be some variation in color use at any age or stage, depending upon the child and his or her experiences. However, on the whole, the stages of normal artistic development are a good place to start in considering how color is used by children and what role emotions may or may not play in that process. An excellent resource for a more in-depth study of color, developmental aspects, and feelings is the work of Golomb (1990).

There has been a great deal of discussion as to the meaning of color usage in drawings specifically with reference to emotion, but this information is rather anecdotal and impressionistic for the most part. For example, red seems to be thought of as the most emotional color, attributed to aggression, anger, and hate, "an issue of vital significance, a burning problem, surging emotions or danger" (Furth, 1988), as well as passion, affection, and expressiveness. Red also seems to be a dominant or preferred color with both older and younger children. Pure yellow has generally been associated with energy, light, and positive feelings, while blue has been related to emotions such as peacefulness or depression, as well as meanings associated with water and sky. The excessive use of black seems to, for the most part, conjure up negative connotations. Furth (1988), in his many years of work with children, notes: "Black may indicate or symbolize the unknown; if used for shading, it is generally seen as negative, projecting 'dark' thoughts, a threat, or fear" (p. 97).

In early research on children's paintings, Alschuler and Hattwick (1947) noted that younger children prefer warm colors such as red and orange, while older children prefer blues and greens, the cool colors. This difference in choice was thought to be due to younger children's natural impulsiveness and older children's developing sense of control. Their studies involved psychoanalytic evaluations of the easel paintings of young children, which, unfortunately, were methodologically flawed (there was a lack of standardization of colors in terms of number and kinds available to the subjects). It also seems that their study sought to support a relationship between the use of color and existing information on the children's behaviors and personality traits, particularly impulse control and conflicts, an emphasis representative of the psychoanalytic thinking of the time.

These are just a few of many speculations as to meanings of colors in children's art expressions. As would be expected, there are also personal meanings and cultural aspects to color. At times, children's use of color seems to contradict and even surprise us as to what we normally expect. For example, one study found that children who are depressed used more color in their works than nondepressed children (Gulbro-Leavitt & Schimmel, 1991), contradicting prevailing beliefs that depressed children use black or monochromatic color schemes. This result is possibly due to chance, but it remains a result that reflects the complexity of understanding children's emotional lives through art expression.

Color use can also be influenced by the task or art activity, complicating understanding of color and emotion. Golomb (1990) notes that in drawing images of a family or human figures, 5-year-olds often use a single color, but when they are asked to draw a garden, multiple colors are more frequently used. It seems that when details such as line and shape become important, color use is subordinated, and when color becomes important to the theme (in this case, a garden, which involves flowers), it is used more frequently by this age group. However, this use of color changes with age, and Golomb (1990) found a great deal of variation from year to year in children's drawings of human figures and gardens. In general, it seems that when children are interested in getting more details into their images, they prefer monochromatic color schemes. Some children may even prefer a pencil, since drawing a person requires complex articulation and it also allows for erasure of any "mistakes." Color, in these cases, may not be an important consideration and cannot be interpreted for emotional significance. Children are also influenced by the current fads in color; for example, purple, the color of the popular character Barney, has recently turned up in many children's art expressions.

Size

One other structural element in drawings that is thought to have emotional significance is the relative size of items, particularly figures. Almost all projective drawing literature concurs that the size of a drawing of a human figure is highly significant, most relating this to a sense of self-esteem or personal adequacy (Buck, 1948; Hammer, 1958; Koppitz, 1968, 1984; Machover, 1949). This belief is based on the assumption that children express themselves symbolically through drawings and that they are creating a self-image reflecting feelings about themselves when asked to draw a human figure. Although very small drawings, especially of human figures, may have a connection to the child's sense of self, there can be other reasons in addition to low self-esteem. For example, one little boy told me that he drew himself very small because "I was very angry at my dad and I wanted to be small to let all the anger out so my dad would not see it" (Figure 5.2). Understandably, he did not want his father, who was physically abusive to his mother and him, to know that he was angry, fearing that his dad might retaliate and, to some extent, feeling guilty that he was mad at his parent. Making himself smaller in his drawing and therefore less threatening or noticeable to the abusive parent was consistent with his other skills at protecting himself from violence. The little girl described in Chapter 2 who drew very a small figure in response to her initial meeting with the art therapist is another good example (Figures 2.4, 2.5, and 2.6): Sometimes children draw small figures simply to hide themselves from adults whom they perceive to be intrusive. Once a relationship and trust are established, the size of figures may dramatically change even in a short amount of time.

"Art Behaviors"

In addition to looking at the art product for emotional content, looking at children's art expressions involves observing their: "art behaviors" (Malchiodi, 1990, 1997); that is, how they react to art directives or drawing tasks. It is important to watch how children use materials

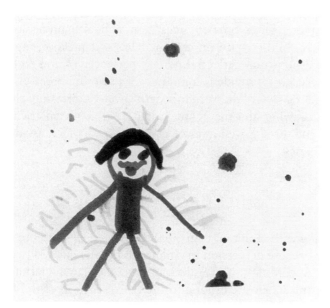

FIGURE 5.2. "I was very angry at my dad and I wanted to be small to let all the anger out so my dad would not see it," drawing by a 7-year-old boy who had been physically abused by his father.

(tentatively, confidently, fearfully, dissociatively, repetitively) in addition to the content of their final products. For example, children who have experienced violence to themselves often remain in state of constant alert and pseudophobia (Silvern, Karyl, & Landis, 1995), fearing recurrence of a previously traumatic experience. A child may be hypervigilent and exhibit a "frozen watchfulness" (Ounstead, Oppenheimer, & Lindsay, 1974) when an imminent personal threat is sensed; this can be triggered by anything characteristic of the original traumatizing events, including sights, sounds, smells, or other experiences. The art process may become a triggering event for recall of trauma, reflecting children's fears and other powerful emotions. Thus, when an abused or traumatized child spills a container of paint, he may be fearful of how the therapist (the authority figure) will respond to his actions. Perhaps spilling a soda at the dinner table caused a parent to become violent to the child, sibling, or spouse. The experience of spilling the paint seems to become a metaphor for what was a precipitant event in creating a scenario for violence in the family system.

Emotional content in children's drawings is often very compelling, and therapists are frequently confronted with expressions of crisis, fear, anxiety, and other painful experiences. The remainder of this chapter focuses on two areas mental health professionals who work with children face on a regular basis: depression and trauma. Art expressions may reflect children's perspectives and feelings and, at the very least, provide a container for powerful emotions associated with crisis. Children can benefit from expressing themselves through drawing and may convey images that reveal their anxiety, despair, and fears as well as more positive aspects such as adaptability and resiliency.

CHILDHOOD DEPRESSION

In working with children, I am often concerned about depression, particularly because depression in children is usually masked by other behaviors. According to the American Psychiatric Association's (1994) most recent diagnostic criteria in the fourth edition of the *Diagnostic and Statistical Manual of Mental Disorders* (DSM-IV), diagnosis of depression in children is essentially the same as for adults. The manner in which depression is manifested in children is, however, debatable.

Some believe that the disorder is similar to adult forms of depression, while others consider it to be masked and displayed through other behavioral problems (Kashini et al., 1981). Depression in children is a component of many other disorders and conditions, making it hard to separate and difficult to identify. For many years children were not believed to be susceptible to depression; now most clinicians agree that many children do experience depression and that it is a serious psychological condition.

Children who are depressed may seem sad or withdrawn, but some may disguise their feelings through other responses and reactions. Typically, depression is apparent in feelings of hopelessness or worthlessness, loss of energy, excessive guilt, or uncontrollable crying. However, young children in particular may not exhibit any of these behaviors, may not appear sad at all, and are overlooked for depression. Other children express depression through anger, irritability, or aggressive behavior, and may be evaluated as having a conduct disorder because they are constantly having difficulties getting along with peers or family. Some children who are depressed may act out their frustrations through hurting animals, pyromania, encopresis, and nocturnal enuresis, uncomfortable expressing their hostility with people.

Therapists naturally look for indications of depression in the children they see and are often hopeful of finding clues to children's depression through their art and play activities in order to be of help. Unfortunately, identifying depression through children's art expressions is not at all easy or foolproof. In fact, it is one of the more difficult aspects to recognize when looking at children's drawings, probably because of the complicated ways that depression manifests itself in children themselves. It is hard for even the most skilled mental health professionals to differentiate among full-blown depression, grief reactions, and sadness in children, and other clues are often needed in addition to what the child draws or depicts to determine what the child is experiencing. However, considering the debilitating effects of depression, it is still important to look at children's art expressions for possible signs. Drawing serves an important purpose for children experiencing depression, since it offers them a way to express their feelings of sadness as well as the anger, anxiety, and frustration that may accompany it. Drawings allow for complex feelings to be expressed and also provide children with an opportunity to convey their personal stories to the helping adult.

PROJECTIVE DRAWING TESTS, ART-BASED ASSESSMENTS, AND DEPRESSION

There are numerous references to depression in projective assessment measures such as the House–Tree–Person (HTP), Kinetic Family Drawing (KFD), and Draw-A-Person (DAP). Most observations point to characteristics such as very small drawings, abnormally light pressure, and lack of detail as indications of depression. The majority of these studies, however, have focused on adults. Wadeson (1971) studied the drawings of depressed adults, noting that when severe depression was present, less color was used, empty space was increased, less effort and investment were shown in the process, and more constricted and less meaningful imagery was included. Since adults were the subject of her study, it is difficult to apply this information to children, although there may be some connections. Gantt (1990) concurred that drawings by depressed patients used less space and fewer details than did normal controls.

The structural elements of children's drawings may be more helpful in identifying depression than making inferences from specific symbols. Gulbro-Levitt and Schimmel (1991) used an adaptation of a drawing assessment tool, the Diagnostic Drawing Series (DDS; Cohen, Hammer, & Singer, 1988) to evaluate structural elements in children's drawings with the goal of assessing depression. Although their findings were inconclusive, they did indicate a trend for the following characteristics: use of one third of the paper, less use of idiosyncratic color, use of more shading and geometric shapes, and the introduction of animals but not people in their drawings. One limitation of the study involved the use of self-rating scales that were assumed to be sensitive enough to identify depression in children. Again, given that depressive symptoms tend to overlap with other diagnoses, this study underscores that detection of depression is often difficult, especially with children.

Silver (1988, 1993) has done extensive work in studying children's images related to depression using Draw-A-Story (DAS), a drawing protocol she developed. A subsequent form of the DAS, the Silver Drawing Test (SDT; Silver, 1996a), also addresses the evaluation of depression as well as cognitive and creative skills. The DAS was designed to screen for depression using a set of simple line drawings created by Silver to stimulate children to develop drawings and stories about their drawings. The set of images was selected because in

Silver's estimation, they seemed to prompt negative fantasies. The actual task involves allowing children to choose two images from the set and asking them to combine these images in a drawing. Children are encouraged to make their drawings in any way they wish and to add details or change characteristics of the original images. The child is then asked to title the picture and to provide a story about the drawing, giving a description of the content in the picture.

For example, Figure 5.3, "The Wedding of the Forest Animals," is a drawing that would be rated as strongly positive according to Silver's scale because both the image and the title indicate a loving relationship. Figure 5.4 is a less positive image titled "The cat wants food and nobody is there to feed her and the dog scared her." This drawing is rated as moderately negative because the main subject of the drawing is frightened and hungry, the environment is hostile, and the outcome of the situation is unclear. Last, Figure 5.5, by a 13-year-old boy, is titled "Prey" and depicts a mouse being eaten by a snake. This drawing conveys a strongly negative theme where the future is hopeless (in this case, for the mouse) and a principal subject is helpless and dying.

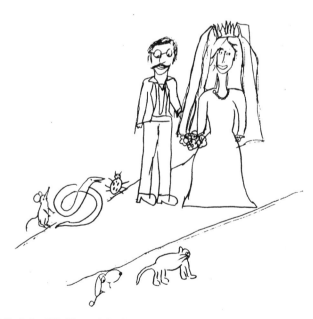

FIGURE 5.3. "Wedding of the Forest Animals," Silver Draw-A-Story by an 11-year-old girl. From *Draw-A-Story: Screening for Depression and Emotional Needs* by Rawley Silver. Copyright 1988 by Rawley Silver. Reprinted by permission.

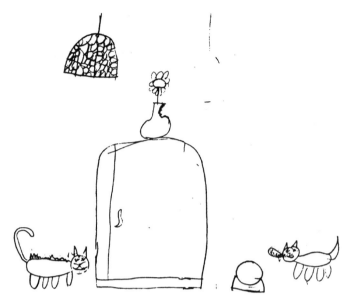

FIGURE 5.4. "The cat wants food and nobody is there to feed her and the dog scared her," Silver Draw-A-Story by an 8-year-old girl. From *Draw-A-Story: Screening for Depression and Emotional Needs* by Rawley Silver. Copyright 1988 by Rawley Silver. Reprinted by permission.

Silver's work is based on the idea that there is a continuum of depression ranging from moderate depression to more severe depression and suicidal and self-destructive thoughts and that these various degrees of depression may be seen in children's DAS tests. According to Silver (1996a), at least three preliminary studies supported that the DAS was useful in determining clinical depression, and two of these studies involved children. Although strongly negative content in the children's drawings did not necessarily indicate depression, and strongly positive content did not exclude depression, the findings suggested that children who respond to the DAS with strongly negative themes may be at a higher risk for depression.

Silver's DAS is an interesting tool in the detection of childhood depression for several reasons. Evaluation of the DAS is based on content or meaning of a drawing, rather than structural elements, such as spacing, color, or line quality in children's drawings. The DAS is also an open-ended activity, allowing children to make choices and offers a degree of freedom of expression. Projective drawing tasks such as the HTP, DAP, or KFD are more specific about what to draw and may be less likely to reveal creative or fantasy material.

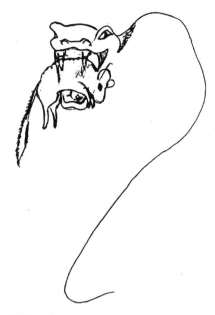

FIGURE 5.5. "Prey," Silver Draw-A-Story by a 13-year-old boy. From *Draw-A-Story: Screening for Depression and Emotional Needs* by Rawley Silver. Copyright 1988 by Rawley Silver. Reprinted by permission.

Silver's drawing protocol and thinking about depression in children support the concept that metaphor and story are important components in understanding and determining if a child is at risk for an affective disorder. Children experience depression in various ways and their own stories about their drawings are particularly useful to understanding what they are feeling when they are depressed. Children's narratives are important to the therapeutic process, particularly when they are in a great deal of emotional pain or have self-destructive tendencies.

THE IMPORTANCE OF THEMES AND NARRATIVES IN ASSESSING DEPRESSION

My own thinking about depression and how children's spontaneous drawings may reveal depression is also based on children's own narratives in response to their images rather than specific elements or symbols in their art expressions. Four themes seem particularly important both in the content of the art expressions and in children's narratives: mourning/bereavement, isolation, despair, and destructive or self-destructive themes. These four aspects, however, are not easily separated, and children often express one or more of them in their drawings and their narratives about their art expressions.

Expressions of *mourning* or *bereavement* are generally easy to recognize in children's artwork. Figure 5.6 is a painting of a black rainbow by a 9-year-old girl who was not outwardly depressed but who had a great deal to be depressed about after experiencing years of physical neglect and abuse and witnessing violence in her home. Her rainbow painting is easy to comprehend, filled with mostly blackness and a little green, overshadowed by a black cloud on the top portion. This use of black in an image most children at her age would make quite colorful is sometimes a direct indicator of existing depression. Other obvious indicators can include tears (Figure 5.7) and rain (Figure 5.8), which may appear in drawings of houses, landscapes, or other environmental themes. These are certainly not always indicative of grief or sadness, but given that they rarely appear in children's drawings, representations of tears or rain should be given attention if a therapist is concerned about possible depression in a child.

Isolation may include feelings of alienation, abandonment, and rejection. At times, themes of isolation in children's drawings are

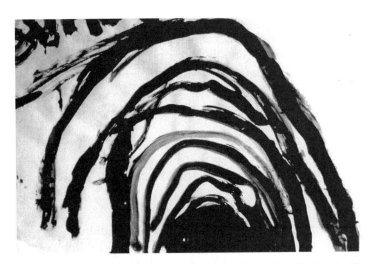

FIGURE 5.6. Painting of a black rainbow by a 9-year-old girl. From *Breaking the Silence* by Cathy A. Malchiodi. Copyright 1997 by Brunner/Mazel. Reprinted by permission.

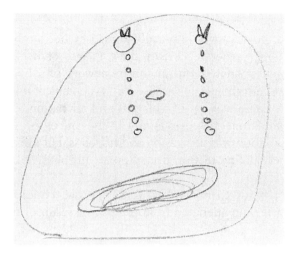

FIGURE 5.7. Drawing of a face with tears by a depressed 8-year-old girl.

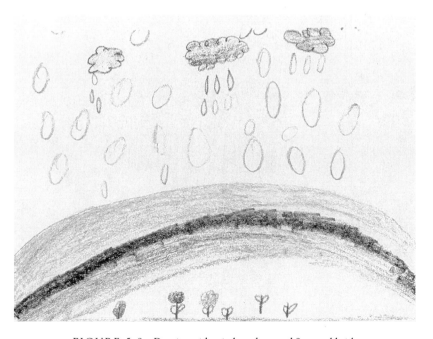

FIGURE 5.8. Drawing with rain by a depressed 8-year-old girl.

quite striking,and other times, they are more subtle. A vivid example, an 8-year-old girl who was physically abused by her mother and her mother's live-in partner repeatedly drew images of herself isolated from others, encapsulated within the framework of a house (Figure 5.9). Physical battering, sexual abuse, or psychological maltreatment may certainly cause feelings of isolation and alienation, especially if the injury comes from one's own family. In the case of this girl, the experience of isolation was depressing and hopeless, but also provided a measure of personal protection from a physically abusive home situation.

It is important to remember that depressed children who are withdrawn or feeling alienated from others as a result of trauma may

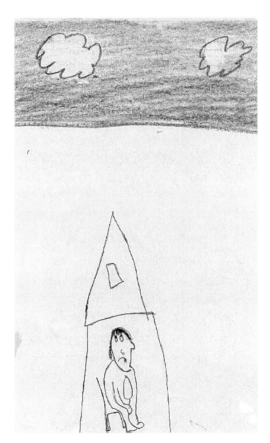

FIGURE 5.9. An 8-year-old girl's image of herself isolated and encapsulated within the framework of a house.

sit mutely in an art therapy group because of psychic numbness or intrusive thoughts and may have a difficult time focusing on drawing tasks because of attention difficulties or dissociation. Children who are depressed often feel hopeless, helpless, and empty. Their feelings of *despair* can be profound and often include guilt for their own feelings, thoughts, or actions. They also may express wishes for changes in their lives, families, or living situations that may be impossible to achieve, thus adding to their sense of hopelessness in the future. A 12-year-old girl whose father was sexually abusive to her and her sister expressed both her sadness and guilt about disclosing the sexual abuse to protective service workers. She shows herself openly grieving, with tears coming down her cheeks and praying for a positive change to take place between her parents now that they were separated because of her disclosure (Figure 5.10). A 9-year-old depressed girl who was sexually abused along with her two sisters by her father, described her feelings of hopelessness that her family would change for the better, saying that her mother was pregnant and "I hope it will be a boy this time. Maybe God will help us because I can't do anything about it. " Her statement expresses her longing to change the family pattern of incest, hoping that a baby brother would not be abused by her father

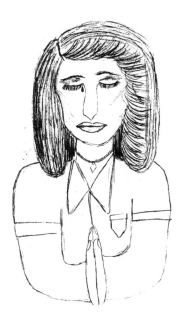

FIGURE 5.10. A 12-year-old girl's image of herself crying and praying.

as were the three sisters. Her drawing is a self-image with an incomplete body and what seems to be an expressionless face (Figure 5.11).

Destructive themes related to depression include self-hatred, self-denigration, self-destruction, guilt, and extremely low self-esteem. Children may take a self-deprecating attitude toward themselves, drawing self-images that make fun of themselves or depict themselves as "ugly" or unattractive. It is not surprising that children who have been neglected or abused view themselves as damaged, freakish, or unattractive in their drawings. For example, an 8-year-old girl who was neglected and abused depicts herself with comical and negative features, titling it "[Girl's name] Is Terrible?" (Figure 5.12).

Other depressed children's drawings may reflect their own self-destructive behaviors and feelings of failure. An 8-year-old boy, Felix, who was placed in a group home for boys because of family problems, was depressed because of separation from his family and school and acted out his frustration through his encopresis. Unfortunately, at first it was difficult to determine which of the boys had this condition, because evidence of the encopresis was found only in public areas of the home (on the walls of the recreation room and in several bathrooms) so no one could identify which boy was leaving and smearing the feces. Although Felix was among several suspects at a group home, no one was quite certain. The staff psychologist asked me if I had any ideas about which boy was doing it, but unfortunately, I was as perplexed as the rest of the staff.

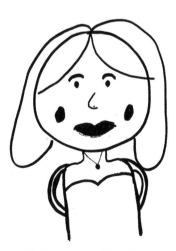

FIGURE 5.11. A 9-year-old girl's drawing of herself. From *Breaking the Silence* by Cathy A. Malchiodi. Copyright 1997 by Brunner/Mazel. Reprinted by permission.

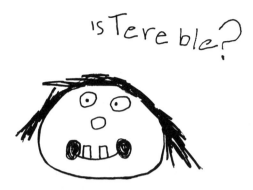

FIGURE 5.12. "[Girl's name] Is Terrible," self-image by an 8-year-old girl.

I decided to call together all the "suspects" to the art room, discussed the problem with them, and then asked them to draw a picture of anything they wanted to draw. Felix drew a well-detailed race car emitting a large plume of black smoke out of the rear tailpipe (Figure 5.13). Although race cars are typical themes that appear in boys' drawings, the black smoke was noticeably profuse. While the smoke could simply be car exhaust, it struck me that it might be representative of another type of exhaust, especially since Felix spent quite some time perfecting it in his picture. After the group, I shared my suspicions with Felix, and he admitted to me that he indeed was the one who was smearing feces throughout the facility. He was not only depressed and frustrated about his family situation, but also about his en-

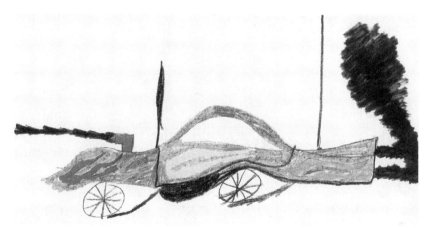

FIGURE 5.13. Eight-year-old Felix's drawing of a race car with exhaust.

copresis, as well as ashamed and embarassed about what he had been doing.

Felix's car exhaust turned out to be a metaphor for his problem, but it is a benign image compared to some more violent imagery one might see from seriously depressed children. Some drawings are much more visually intense in content and may be indicative of extreme rage directed at others or at the self (Figure 5.14). Self-destructive imagery brings with it concerns for suicide, even in children. Suicide threats are always serious circumstances and can occur with children who are depressed. Although the number of suicides in latency age children is relatively low, the rate has increased over time (Pfeffer, 1986) and is of clinical concern. Fortunately, most children are less

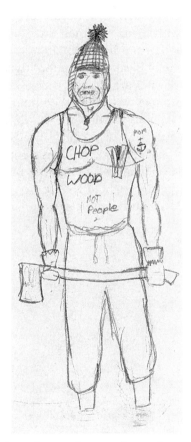

FIGURE 5.14. "Murderer," drawing of a man with an ax by a preadolescent boy with depression and conduct disorder.

isolated than adults, have greater emotional support, and are thus not as likely to complete or carry out a suicidal attempt. However, although infrequent, suicide threats are important to consider in light of children's depression.

Children's suicide threats often come as a gesture or attempt to change what are frightening or unacceptable situations. Mike, an 8-year-old boy who was physically abused by both his mother and his mother's numerous live-in boyfriends, decided one day to stand in a second story window and threaten to jump into the courtyard below. Staff and the facility's therapists were able to coax him out of the window to safety, although he made it clear that he would not speak to his mother. In work with his therapist immediately after the attempt, he drew a small image of a face with what he said was a screaming mouth (Figure 5.15). He was very anxious while creating the drawing, possibly because he realized how close he had come to either seriously hurting himself or ending his life. The simplicity of the drawing very effectively captures his fright, anxiety, and confused feelings about the incident.

What becomes most important about the content of this drawing is the child's meaning or intention of a suicide threat. In looking at this particular image as a "cry for help" or message of deep despair and desperation, it is important to determine to whom this message is directed. In this case, the message was directed to the mother who was herself abusive and allowed her son to be abused by others and also to the staff to intervene on the boy's behalf. In asking him what the person depicted in the drawing wanted to say, Mike said simply that "the person's mother would be very, very sorry that the boy died."

Evidence of suicide intent in drawings like depression is often

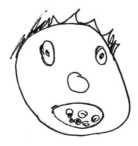

FIGURE 5.15. Eight-year-old Mike's drawing of himself after suicide attempt. From *Breaking the Silence* by Cathy A. Malchiodi. Copyright 1997 by Brunner/Mazel. Reprinted by permission.

difficult to pinpoint with any accuracy in art expressions. Mike's drawings prior to his suicide attempt, for example, indicated his frustration with his family situation and his poor sense of self, and but no obvious intent or plans to carry out a suicide were evident. In fact, in the days before his attempt, he was outwardly very positive and responsive to those around him.

Cox (1984) in her work with depressed and suicidal child, adolescent, and adult clients proposed 10 themes of self-destruction in art expressions that may be helpful to therapists in determining if a child is depressed from looking at the child's drawings over time and may serve as warning of suicide risk:

> 1) *anger*, hostility, aggression, rage; 2) *self-hatred*, self-accusation, self-denigration, self-destruction, guilt, extremely low self-esteem; 3) *despair*, hopelessness, helplessness, suffering, emptiness, resignation; 4) *alienation*, rejection, abandonment, isolation, loss of or fear of loss of a significant other, extreme vulnerability; 5) hostile interpersonal relations; 6) *frustrated need for dependency*, early deprivation; 7) *longing for spiritual rebirth*, for restitution, for reunion with loved one; 8) *tension*, anxiety, frustration, feelings of impending chaos, increased impulsivity; 9) *fragmentation*, disintegration, depersonalization; 10) *ambivalence toward death*. (p. 44)

Cox hypothesized that five or more indicators in art expressions over time might constitute sufficient evidence for serious consideration of potential self-destructive behaviors. Although Cox's proposed themes resulted from work with both children and adults, they are still helpful guidelines when one is looking at children's drawings for content that is possibly predictive of depression or suicidal tendencies.

TRAUMA

Children's experiences of trauma have received increased attention from healthcare professionals due to heightened awareness of the effects of domestic violence, physical and sexual abuse, street violence, and catastrophic events. Traumatized children experience a wide range of emotions and profound psychological pain including anxiety, helplessness, fear, loneliness, depression, vulnerability, and despair. Loss is also a central issue in any type of trauma and may be related to the deprivation of a parent or significant other because of divorce, imprisonment, mental or physical illness, or death. Children may also react traumatically to a parent's unemployment or to moving to a new residence, neighborhood, or state. Multiple losses are quite common in any traumatic circumstance and can impact children in a variety of ways.

According to DSM-IV (American Psychiatric Association, 1994), symptoms of posttraumatic stress disorder (PTSD) include a loss in ability to enjoy previously enjoyed activities, constricted affect, a foreshortened sense of the future, somatic complaints, fear of repeated trauma, and possible "psychic numbness" after the trauma. Hypervigilance, anxiety, withdrawal, recurrent nightmares, and declines in cognitive performance are also common to PTSD (Terr, 1990; Green, 1983). The term "PTSD" was originally applied to survivors of natural disasters, war experiences, and accidents who experienced such symptoms. It is now commonly understood that children who have been exposed to violence, particularly any type of family violence or physical abuse, may also experience posttraumatic stress disorder (American Psychiatric Association, 1994). Although it is a diagnosis historically given to adults, PTSD has been cited as a possible outcome of abuse in children (Pynoos & Eth, 1985; Green, 1983; Anthony, 1986; Webb, 1991) and can occur at any age during childhood.

Children use art expression to express trauma and associated feelings of grief, mourning and loss and often master trauma through play activity or artistic expression. Alice Miller (1986), author of many contemporary writings on the trauma of child abuse, notes the connections between her own childhood abuse and artistic creativity. She observes that feelings resulting from childhood trauma take tangible form in art expressions:

> The repressed feelings of my childhood—the fear, despair, and utter loneliness—emerged in my pictures, and at first I was all alone with the task of working these feelings through. For at that point I didn't know any painters with whom I would have been able to share my new found knowledge of childhood, nor did I have any colleagues to whom I could have explained what was happening to me when I painted. I didn't want to be given psychoanalytic interpretations, didn't want to hear explanations offered in terms of Jungian symbols. I wanted only to let the child in me speak and paint long enough for me to understand her language. (p. 7)

As a child in Poland during World War II, Nelly Toll began to keep a diary of her experiences, using words and images. In her more recent memoir (1993) she writes:

> Paintings . . . provided me with an escape into a fantasy world. I painted over sixty watercolors, made up cheerful tales about them, and sewed pictures and stories together into small booklets with white thread; through the magic of art, I became part of that happy world of illusion. The five-by-seven-inch and seven-by-ten inch sheets of paper were filled with colorful flowers, blue skies, loving adults, and carefree children busy with normal daily activities. Only symbolically did they reflect my feelings of apprehension about the constant danger surrounding us. (pp. ix–x)

Although describing the meaning of art for her from an adult perspective, Toll's words speak strongly to the importance of art expression for children during times of stress, crisis, and trauma. For Toll, art making was a secret world filled with bright colors and images that seemed to illustrate a world for the most part untouched by the horrors of what was taking place around her. However, through her images she was able express her underlying fears, pain, and outrage of profoundly terrifying events she was experiencing during World War II. Her drawings and paintings became a way to record life's beauty in the face of overwhelming circumstances, a lifeline to stability, a place for wishes and fantasies, and a connection to humanity in the face of inhumanity.

Toll's images and her poignant observations also make an important point: Art represents a unique viewpoint or individual way of dealing with trauma for each child. Her work also underscores the diversity of expression by children who may have been traumatized. Art, in contrast to serving as a mirror of crises or pain, is also a way to express dreams of what might have been and to escape from horrors and experiences sometimes too difficult to express in other ways.

For children who have been traumatized by family violence, abuse, or other crises, drawings may become visual fantasies for something that is impossible or unreachable. Joanne, an 8-year-old girl from an abusive family, consistently drew images of home environments that she rarely experienced. These drawings often contained pleasant scenes and included colorful houses with gardens and toys (Figure 5.16). She often described these drawings as pictures of stable and nurturing home environments where she and her family could live in long enough to grow vegetables, something she longed for but did not have at the time. In reality, Joanne was often depressed and upset with her mother who was a substance abuser who moved from abusive relationship to relationship, and, in the past, had been abusive to Joanne and her younger brother. In many ways, Joanne's life was similiar to that of survivors of war or upheaval because she was constantly faced with turmoil and violence in her own home. Drawing was one way to create a more positive worldview as well as hope for her family's future.

Art expression seems to be well suited as a modality with children in trauma because it may be easier for them to use visual modes of communication before being able to talk about trauma (Malchiodi, 1990, 1997; Stronach-Buschel, 1990). However, as shown, children express their trauma in somewhat different ways. Although there are a number of commonalities in the structure and contents of images created in response to trauma or crisis, each child responds through art expression in a personal way. For example, traumatic events may be expressed by

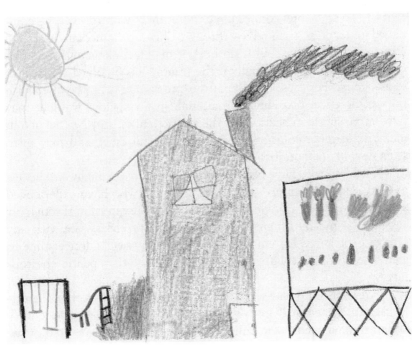

FIGURE 5.16. Drawing of a happy home by Joanne, an 8-year-old girl from an abusive family.

children in both fully-formed images or in sparse renderings; some children will express the horror of their experiences in great detail, whereas others may prefer to give as few details as possible.

Differences in art expression can be a function of the situation, that is, whether the child is supported by family, friends, or others or trusts the therapist enough to express freely and safely; of whether he or she has the ability to communicate artistically (e.g., some children have innate capacities to express through art, while others may be less talented or interested); and developmental aspects (e.g., the age and developmental level of the young artist) can affect the content, details, and style. The type and duration of trauma will inevitably have an impact on the art expression; for example, the experience of a tornado, something that is perceived to be beyond one's control and random, will be different from the expression of family violence or abuse. It is important for therapists to remember that it is a difficult task for a child to take a pencil or crayon and depict a traumatic memory and often one that children do not initiate spontaneously for reasons of fear, personal safety, secrecy, or denial.

Personal responses to crisis also will have an effect on the content of the art expression. Some children may wish or even be compelled to express themselves through drawing immediately after a traumatic experience. But for others, it may feel dangerous to depict what has happened, especially if the trauma has involved physical or sexual abuse. For these children, art expression may not be filled with horror, violence, or traumatic material, in an obvious way but may have more subtle indications of their experiences, may be couched in metaphoric representations rather than literal ones, and may even seem devoid of emotional content.

Children who have been chronically traumatized may also be less able to express themselves freely, while those who have experienced acute trauma (i.e., a single incident) may find expression through art easier. Chronically traumatized children may feel less safe with any type of expression, including art, and they may need a longer time to gain a sense of trust with the therapist and the therapeutic environment.

Art expression may serve as a way to integrate parts of the identity that are temporarily lost or confused when trauma is experienced. When trauma occurs, the child may be left feeling fragmented or see the world in a fragmented way. The trauma is a line of demarcation distinguishing a time of relative safety and a time of distress, fear, anxiety, and other concerns associated with experiencing the trauma. What seems to be common is that most children, despite their experiences with painful events, will still find joy in the act of creating art. It may be that through creation of art there is a natural experience of wholeness or working toward wholeness and this, in and of itself, may be what is most important to understand about traumatized children's drawings and their importance in therapy.

CHILD ABUSE AND EXPOSURE TO FAMILY OR SOCIETAL VIOLENCE

Many therapists expect that the art expressions of children traumatized by violence will be vivid and expressive and will depict detailed scenes of domestic violence or abuse. As shown earlier, however, in many cases children do not spontaneously draw the traumatizing event, and most children seem to include rather sparse details in terms of structural elements, line quality, and content. Colors used are often limited, and children may predominantly use black and/or red in their drawings (Malchiodi, 1990, 1997). Children who are traumatized by violence or abuse may quickly execute an image, dedicating little attention to detail and drawing poorly integrated or composed figures. Their art expressions are simplistic, often resembling stereotyped cartoons or doodles (Terr, 1981, 1990; Malchiodi, 1990, 1997).

This lack of content, detail, and color is not surprising for several reasons. First, children who come from violent homes, have been exposed to street violence or other abusive situations may be withdrawn or frightened, or they may be disassociated from life around them. When a child is psychologically exhausted, the robustness of the expression is often affected: The child simply does not have the internal resources to represent on paper what has been a complicated and exhausting series of traumatic events. Depression may take its toll, leaving children little energy or tolerance for art expression or causing them to be withdrawn and uninterested in sharing much about their feelings, even though art is generally an enjoyable and motivating activity. Children may feel disconnected from their own capacity for expression and, in some cases, may be very defended in their spontaneous expressions, particularly when asked to make a drawing about a theme directly related to their trauma. For example, when asked to make an image of a family, many children who have been abused by a family member or who feel protective of their family situation may not comply with the request or may draw simplistic or stereotypic renditions in order to comply with the request. They may feel threatened and unsafe within the therapeutic relationship, fearing that they will expose a family secret or express something that will compromise themselves with a perpetrator.

Children exposed to extreme societal violence may also exhibit the effects of trauma in both their behaviors and their art expressions. Tibbetts (1989), in his work with children from Northern Ireland, used drawing to help children express themselves and to begin the process of working through traumatic violence. Tibbetts began with a brief and supportive discussion of the child's traumatizing experience, asking children to draw a picture of anything they would like and tell a story about their pictures. Although the children were not specifically asked to draw a picture related to their traumas, most children drew images related to or depicting their traumatizing events (Figure 5.17).

The children in Tibbetts's study generally used minimal details in their drawings to visually describe the trauma, feelings, or impressions; used a constricted focus (i.e., a lack of background detail in order to more fully focus on the traumatizing event); or did not integrate the background with the actual event. Tibbetts (1989) observed that "the majority of children demonstrated a flat and generally depressed affect during the post-drawing interviews, and actively resisted the interviewer's attempts to elicit their feelings about the traumatizing event" (p. 94). He noted that these children were subjected to an environment that encourages violence and promotes constant persistent trauma and anxiety, which is perhaps why these children had more difficulty in sharing or releasing emotions than children who had not been exposed to extreme violence.

Repetition seems to be present in both the structural elements and the art behaviors of children who come from violent homes, who have experienced abuse, and who have witnessed violent acts. Children may repeat images related to the trauma they have experienced, or may repeat themes of rescue (such as the police or firemen coming), or violence and destructive acts (aimed at an aggressor or perpetrator) through their art and play activities. For example, a 6-year-old boy repeated a drawing of his house where his physical abuse from his father took place. His narratives about the house drawings were always the same: His father was in the house and would die in a fire, ex-

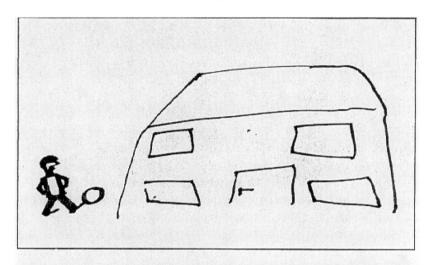

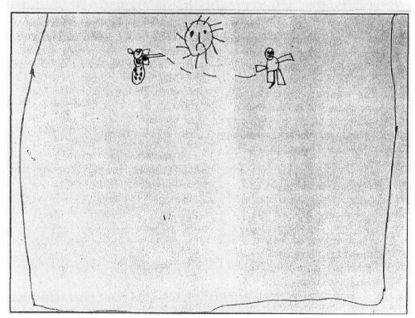

FIGURE 5.17. Drawings by two children from Northern Ireland. From "Characteristics of Artwork in Children with Posttraumatic Stress Disorder in Northern Ireland" by Terry Tibbetts, in *Art Therapy: Journal of the American Art Therapy Association*, 6(3), 92–98. Copyright 1989 by the American Art Therapy Association, Inc. All rights reserved. Reprinted by permission.

plosion, or other disaster that would make escape impossible. The drawings often became unrecognizable because of the maze of lines that evolved along with his stories of destroying his abusive parent (Figure 5.18). A 7-year-old handicapped boy who had experienced the Los Angeles riots in 1992 depicted himself crying while a "bad man" set his house on fire, repeating layers of colors throughout the drawing (Figure 5.19). These repetitions may serve a purpose in the healing process in that they may allow the child to gain a symbolic power over the trauma through repeating an image over and over in art. Although a story may be repeated, children may also repeat a drawing of a simple image or shape or engage in repetitious mark-making or staccato movements of pencil or crayon to paper.

One structural quality that therapists who work with traumatized children, particularly those who have experienced abuse or violence, often wonder about is the meaning of excessive shading in children's drawings. Much of the projective drawing literature connects excessive shading in drawings to anxiety (Hammer, 1958; Machover, 1949). Certainly, it takes quite a bit of energy for a child to vigorously shade a drawing, and excessive shading has turned up as a characteristic of drawings by traumatized children. Epperson (1990) for example,

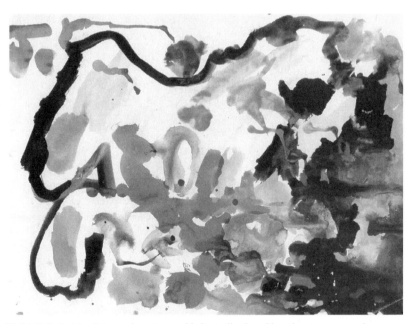

FIGURE 5.18. Painting by a 6-year-old physically abused boy showing a maze of repetitive lines.

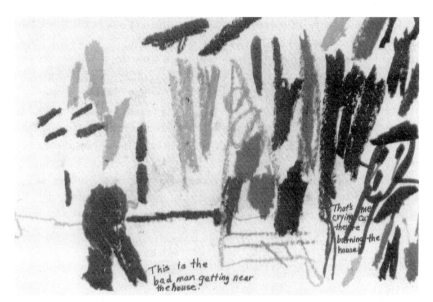

FIGURE 5.19. Drawing by a 7-year-old handicapped boy depicting himself crying while a "bad man" sets his house on fire. From "Art Captures the Impact of the Los Angeles Crisis" by Shirley Riley, in *Art Therapy: Journal of the American Art Therapy Association*, 9(3), 133–144. Copyright 1992 by the American Art Therapy Association, Inc. All rights reserved. Reprinted by permission.

found that in studying children exposed to violence that there was a tendency to shade drawings of the environment, although not to a significant level. However, shading may serve a different psychological purpose rather than pathological or solely indicative of anxiety. For example, some children simply like to fill in their entire drawing with shading, enjoying coloring in the entire page or remembering an art teacher's advice to fill in the whole paper with color. Some children who are traumatized seem to find shading sections of their drawings comforting and sometimes even hypnotic. Excessive shading often serves a function of self-soothing through filling in space in a repetitive way and may be one reason why repetitive activity is often present in traumatized children's art and play activity (Terr, 1990; Malchiodi, 1997).

Although not the major focus of this section, children whose parent, relative, or close friend dies experience trauma, whether or not they witnessed the death of the individual. This type of trauma is similar to that experienced by children from violent homes, those victimized by violence or abuse, or those subjected to catastrophic disas-

ters. Steele, Ginns-Gruenberg, and Lemerand (1995) note that children who lose a loved one have reactions similar to those with PTSD,
including depression, anger, hypervigilance, startle reactions, fears,
and forgetfulness. Therapists working with children grieving the
death of a family member, significant other, or friend may see some of
the characteristics mentioned in this chapter, particularly repetition
of images, limited color range, and narratives and images of grief, isolation, despair, and self-destruction. However, it is important to remember that each child will experience and express loss differently,
and developmental factors as well as the type of loss experienced (e.g.,
sudden death, violent death, death of a parent, death of a friend) will
affect the style and content of children's art expressions.

SEXUAL ABUSE

The experience of sexual abuse, either by a family member or other
individual, is associated with severe emotional effects on children. A
loss of enjoyment in life, lack of affect, a foreshortened sense of the future, somatic complaints, fears of repeated abuse, hypervigilance, anxiety, withdrawal, recurrent nightmares, and declines in cognitive performance are all reported behaviors. Intrusive symptoms such as flash-
backs to the abuse, repetitive thoughts, detachment and numbing,
and in some cases, dissociation (Briere, 1992) are more prominent in
sexual abuse than in other types of trauma and may be more long-
term. There are also additional feelings, including shame, guilt, and
stigmatization.

Because of the profound impact of sexual abuse on children and
because child victims often do not want to disclose or discuss their
abuse, drawings have been repeatedly examined for possible structural
elements and content that may be indicative of sexual abuse and children's perception of it. Although many similar characteristics and
themes have been observed in the drawings of sexually abused children, there seem to be no easily defined or definite list of indicators.
This is not surprising, since each child's experience of abuse is different, dependent on the duration and frequency of abuse, the age of the
child, the perpetrator, and the type of sexual abuse experienced. However, there are some characteristics that suggest sexual trauma may
have occurred and that further investigation and intervention are
warranted on behalf of the child.

One of the stronger indicators is the inclusion of strongly sexual themes or imagery in the children's drawings. Many authors have observed the inclusion of genitalia and/or "private parts" as a possible indicator of sexual abuse (Kelley, 1984, 1985; Yates, Buetler, & Crago, 1985; Hibbard, Roghmann, & Hoekelman, 1987; Faller, 1988; Malchiodi, 1990, 1997). DiLeo (1973), a pediatrician who reviewed thousands of children's drawings, was impressed by the rarity of any portrayal of genitals and associates such portrayal with behavioral disorders, noting that children may not see genitals as being important to their pictures or may omit them because of cultural taboos. Koppitz (1984) also notes that children in our Western culture rarely depict genitals and such depiction is more frequent in children with emotional problems.

Sexual connotation in the drawings of sexually abused children may occur in other ways than portrayal of genitals or nude human figures. Children may also make human figure drawings that display excessive inclusion of sexy dress, an emphasized tongue (Drachnik, 1994) (Figure 5.20), excessive make-up, or long eyelashes or other features that convey seductiveness. Figure 5.21, a pencil drawing by a 10-year-old girl who was sexually abused by her father and who came to a battered women's shelter with her mother and brother, provides an example of sexual connotation. The girl's drawing depicts an extremely sexy woman with an hour-glass figure and sensual cleavage. Although the girl displayed no signs of seductive or inappropriate sexual behavior, her drawings typically included sensual characteristics

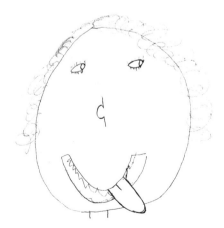

FIGURE 5.20. Drawing with an emphasized tongue by an 8-year-old sexually abused girl.

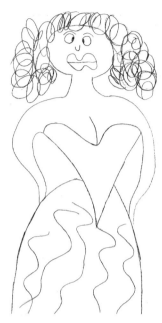

FIGURE 5.21. Drawing by a 10-year-old sexually abused girl. From *Breaking the Silence* by Cathy A. Malchiodi. Copyright 1997 by Brunner/Mazel. Reprinted by permission.

like the ones shown here. She also drew pictures that contained what might be considered "phallic" images, such as a drawing of bees with very large "stingers" going to their beehive (Figure 5.22), identifying the bee's stings as "painful in her behind."

It may be argued that sexual connotations in the art expressions of children may not in themselves indicate sexual abuse. To some extent, children will create images that may have a sexual nature about them. For example, Figure 5.23, a drawing by a 6-year-old boy, shows a figure of a person with breasts, a possibly sexually connotative and thus a suspicious indicator. However, this boy had not been sexually abused; rather, he was fascinated by his mother's breast-feeding of his new baby brother. This fascination with the female breast and issues of nurturance and maternal attention may have been largely responsible for this drawing. DiLeo (1973) observed that in drawings that include a penis, the child may have recently undergone surgery of the genitals (circumcision or hernia operation). Trauma to the body, such as surgery, can bring attention to the area of concern, and children may include and emphasize that body area in their art expression. The

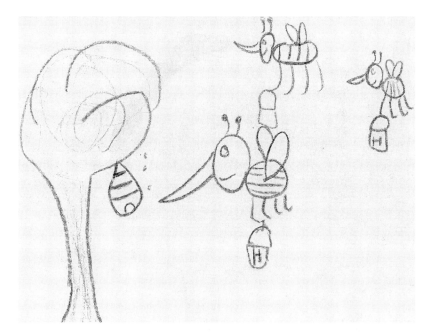

FIGURE 5.22. Drawing by the same 10-year-old girl of bees and stingers that are "painful in her behind."

influence of media in contemporary society may contribute to the drawing of sexual characteristics at an early age, and the accessibility of sexual content and themes through television may have some effect on how children express through visual art (see Chapter 6). It is speculation that television programming has an effect on art expression, but given the prominence of sexual themes on television, videos, and movies, this influence cannot be completely ruled out.

An incomplete body image is another characteristic consistently noted in human figure drawings by sexually abused children (Kelley, 1984; Cohen & Phelps, 1985; Malchiodi, 1997). When requested to draw a person or when spontaneously drawing a person, children who have been sexually abused may only draw a head (as in Figure 5.24) or draw the upper half of the body (as in Figure 5.25). The latter form may appear as a figure in a window or behind some object, such as a car, thus obscuring the lower body half. Kelley (1984) also noted that sexually abused children may draw people with emphasis on their upper portions. This emphasis can include great detail on the face and clothing on the upper body portion, whereas the lower portion is neglected.

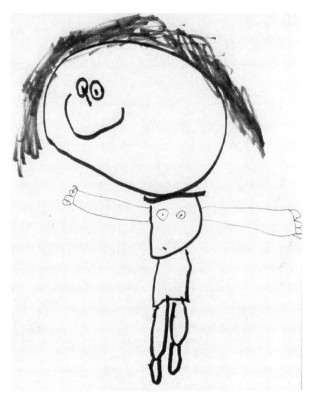

FIGURE 5.23. Drawing of a figure with breasts by a 6-year-old boy. From *Breaking the Silence* by Cathy A. Malchiodi. Copyright 1997 by Brunner/Mazel. Reprinted by permission.

There may be a degree of disorganization of body parts in the art expressions of children who have been sexually abused. Drawings of human figures may appear to be developmentally regressed, are not well-articulated, or may have ambivalent features; in other words, it is difficult to tell what particular features represent. Some children who have been sexually abused may have difficulty drawing a human figure at all because body image is a sensitive topic for them because of the trauma they have experienced. Also, the request to draw a person may elicit some regressive artistic behavior that causes the drawing to appear disorganized. Figure 5.26, a self-portrait by a 6-year-old boy appears very little like a human figure drawing at all and more like pure kinesthetic activity. The boy had been sexually abused by his mother and described his image as "having blood all over it." His other drawings were well-formed, age-appropriate, and more recog-

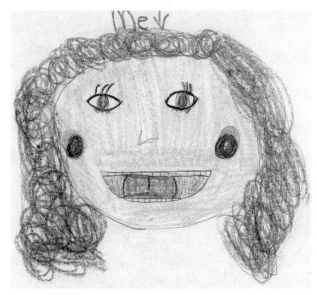

FIGURE 5.24.   Drawing of head without a body by an 8-year-old sexually abused girl.

nizable than his portrait drawing, which seemed to arouse anxiety and loss of control.

A 13-year-old girl who was repeatedly sexually abused by her mother's many "boyfriends," possibly since the age of 6, often drew body images whose components were difficult to identify. Figure 5.27 is a drawing of a person entitled "Cavewoman," drawn by the girl when she was 12 years old. She drew a body that appears to be missing part of its torso and has a foreshortened arm on the right side. The affect of the expression is unsettling, not only because of the distortions to the body but also because of the vacant eyes, rigid torso lining, and cotton-like feet. A second drawing of a person (Figure 5.28) drawn by the girl at age 13 is developmentally regressed and has additional distortions. It is difficult to tell if arms are suggested by the lines at the shoulders and the body is crudely drawn with little detailing. When asked to identify and describe the drawing, the girl's verbal response was as minimal and unidentifiable as her drawing. In her case, it was surmised that she was becoming seriously disturbed and possibly dissociative, the outcome of many years of sexual abuse without resolution or mastery of trauma.

This particular type of disorganization in drawings may occur in

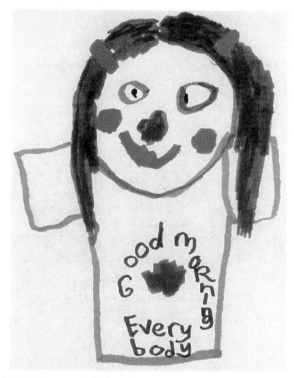

FIGURE 5.25. Drawing of a body without a lower half by a 9-year-old sexually abused girl.

those children whose abuse has been chronic since early childhood, indicating the manifestation of a serious personality disorder. It is reasonable to assume that long-term trauma could dramatically alter the content and style of art expression beyond what would be normally expected.

Other characteristics that have been related to sexual abuse are the inclusion of heart-shaped imagery, developmentally regressive drawing styles, and themes of self-deprecation or self-hate (Cohen & Phelps, 1985; Malchiodi, 1997). Although these and other features and themes have been linked to sexual abuse, they are characteristics that can also be found in drawings of children who have not been sexually abused. However, because of the seriousness of sexual abuse and the probability that many children will not verbally disclose sexual abuse, it is important to consider visual clues in drawings, particularly those mentioned in this section.

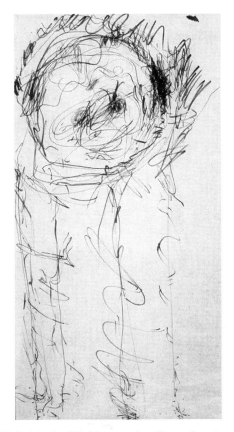

FIGURE 5.26. Scribbled drawing of a self-image by a 6-year-old boy.

DISSOCIATIVE DISORDER

Profound trauma such as sexual abuse may predispose both children and adults to dissociative identity disorder (DID). Symptoms of dissociation include: disengaging from the immediate environment, especially during times of stress, in the form of daydreaming or "spacing out;" emotional numbing; amnesia concerning abuse; and multiple personalities. It is thought that both child and adult survivors reduce or escape their severe emotional pain and trauma through these behaviors, thus allowing them to function in the world.

Traditionally, it has been difficult to assess dissociation in children because it is developmentally normal for children to dissociate to some extent, particularly at the age of 5 or 6 years when children cre-

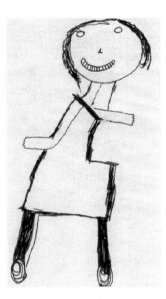

FIGURE 5.27. Self-image by 12-year-old girl who was chronically sexually abused. From *Breaking the Silence* by Cathy A. Malchiodi. Copyright 1997 by Brunner/Mazel. Reprinted by permission.

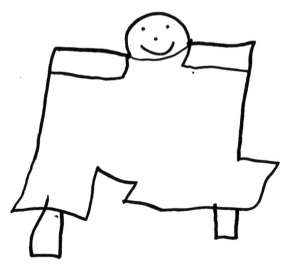

FIGURE 5.28. Self-image by the same girl at age 13. From *Breaking the Silence* by Cathy A. Malchiodi. Copyright 1997 by Brunner/Mazel. Reprinted by permission.

ate imaginary companions and may freely go in and out of fantasy beliefs and stories. Normal dissociative behaviors are thought to decline by age 11 as the child matures and learns to separate reality from imagination. More recently, considerable attention has been given to dissociation in children (Putnam, Guroff, Silberman, Barban, & Post, 1986; Putnam, 1989), and most clinicians who work with trauma agree that dissociative behaviors are present in many children who have been sexually abused.

Some of the possible graphic characteristics of dissociative phenomena in art expression have already been mentioned as general indicators of possible sexual abuse. For example, artistic regression (e.g., drawing that seems to fit different developmental levels) may indicate that a child is switching between dissociative states; in adults with dissociative identity disorder, this movement between developmental levels of artistic expression may signal the appearance of various alters (i.e., personalities) (Cohen & Cox, 1995). A child who has experienced sexual abuse may develop increasingly more distinct multiple personalities over time in order to keep the painful feelings and memories sealed off from consciousness. In older children, this phenomenon may become apparent in art expressions, particularly when developmental levels of expression change frequently, and stylistic changes in images occur. It is important to remember that it is more difficult to assess the meaning of artistic regression with children than adults because, as previously noted, children will often move between developmental levels of artistic expression in their creative activity; a measure of regression is often part of the creative process. However, any repeated regression or movement between levels in a child's drawings is a characteristic worth noting and giving further consideration.

It has been observed that children displaying a high degree of dissociative behavior use art to "self-soothe," often using repetitive lines, marks, and dots in drawing, meshing and blending of colors in paint, or repetitive stabbing or other motions with clay (Sobol & Cox, 1992; Malchiodi, 1994). The therapist may also notice that children have a "far away look" in their eyes and seem as though they are not present to their surroundings. During creative activity, children who dissociate may seem to shift consciousness and not be aware of their environment, probably in an attempt to escape from intrusive memories or emotions. However, it is often difficult to judge whether this is truly a function of dissociation or the preoccupation with the art making process which allows the child a measure of escape from a

world that is troubling or anxiety-producing. Art activity often provides for retreat from reality, and when one is absorbed by creative
process, adult or child, the person will seem to lose all contact with
the world around.

The expression of dissociative identity disorder in adults' art has
been studied more comprehensively for graphic indicators of multiple
personality, resulting in a 10-category list of descriptors (Cohen & Cox,
1995). Until there is more definitive information available on the presentation of childhood dissociation in art expressions, therapists are referred to the texts available on adult art expressions for more information on the possible characteristics of DID in children's drawings.

CATASTROPHIC EVENTS

Natural disasters are obviously traumatic events for everyone, including children. Each child, however, experiences a catastrophic event
differently, depending on the type of disaster and the consequences to
the child, his or her family, and home. Children in natural disasters
may witness buildings on fire or see their homes destroyed, see people
mutilated or killed, or lose parents, siblings, family members, animals,
or friends. There is often a sense or experience of great oss, especially
if one has lost a loved one, beloved pet, or home because of the event.
Children also have concerns about the future, particularly safety for
themselves or their family. At times, children may become angry or
frustrated at parents or caretakers who did not rescue them or did not
arrive in time to protect them. Depending on how the individual
child reacts to the disaster, the impact of the disaster on the self, family, home, and neighborhood, and past experiences with trauma and
loss, children's drawings are diverse in both content and style. Past
losses and trauma are particularly potent and often reemerge with a
new crisis; for example, the traumatic loss several years previous of a
family member may spontaneously appear in images related to the current crisis.

Most agree that natural disasters have a powerful impact on children and that there are both long- and short-term emotional effects
on their art expressions. Herl (1992) notes that children who experienced the Andover Tornado in Kansas in 1991 continued to draw tor-
nado-like images for many weeks after the actual event, and others
drew imaginary beings that helped tornado victims or fought torna-

does. Some observe that children continue to process the trauma effects of natural disasters for a long time period after the event occurred. In her work with children who experienced the Los Angeles
earthquake in 1994, Roje (1995) noticed, even after several months,
children expressed their continuing need for support at termination of
therapy by drawing negative images such as sharks, snakes, and guns,
at times directing their frustration at the therapists. For children who
have had previous traumatic experiences, signs of emotional distress
in their drawings may continue for longer periods than in the drawings of children who have not experienced serious or severe trauma.

Children utilize drawing to express their experience of catastrophic events in several ways. For some, drawing is simply a way to
gain symbolic control over overwhelming circumstances and to establish an inner sense of security and safety in the wake of a catastrophic
event. They may carefully construct their drawings, sometimes even
asking the therapist for a ruler to make perfectly straight lines. Children may also try to "fix" their homes and families through creative
activity, making representations that reflect not only the precarious-
ness of the natural disaster they experienced but also imagining ways
to cope with the circumstances through art expression. A 7-year-old
boy carefully drew a picture of his house with a large crack in the wall,
fearing that if it were not strong enough it would collapse in an after-
shock (Figure 5.29). The boy's deliberate drawing of the house provided an experience of control in the face of the devastation of his home
(Roje, 1995). Some children may refuse to draw at all after the experience of a natural disaster and may be emotionally numb because of
trauma. Roje (1995) notes that some children who experienced the
1994 Los Angeles earthquake declined to talk or draw pictures about
the experience, saying that they "were not scared." These children
chose to play favorite and familiar games or to draw pleasant pictures
that depicted predisaster times, perhaps to escape memories of their
traumatic experiences.

Again, children may regress to developmentally earlier styles of
drawing; for example, a 7-year-old child may feel more comfortable
scribbling or engaging in what Kramer calls precursory activities,
rather than producing a developmentally appropriate image (i.e.,
schematic stage). Like children traumatized by violence or abuse, children who experience catastrophic events may use repetitive patterns
or repeat images to establish a sense of control. For example, a 5-year-
old boy who experienced the 1994 Los Angeles earthquake continued

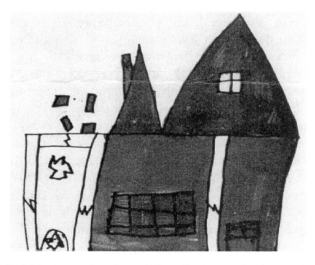

FIGURE 5.29. Drawing by a 7-year-old boy of his house with a large crack in it after the Los Angeles earthquake. From "LA '94 Earthquake in Eyes of Children: Art Therapy with Elementary School Children Who Were Victims of Disaster" by Jasenka Roje, in *Art Therapy: Journal of the American Art Therapy Association*, *12*(4), 237–243. Copyright 1995 by the American Art Therapy Association, Inc. All rights reserved. Reprinted by permission.

to draw the same pattern of lines and circles, even when asked to draw a different picture (Figure 5.30). Repeating a familiar pattern may reinforce a sense of safety for some children, while others may simply perseverate in response to crisis.

As previously mentioned, trauma may have an effect on children's color choices, including those children who have experienced natural disasters. In response to the 1988 Armenian earthquake, Gregorian, Azarian, DeMaria, and McDonald (1996) noted that children who were traumatized by the event became "very restrained in their color choices" (p. 2). Most children only used two or three colors (black or red predominated), did not use mixed colors, and preferred to use only white paper as the background for their art expressions (Figure 5.31). These color choices were not the result of chance. When the therapist removed the black markers, black crayons, black watercolors, and pencils before the children came to the art therapy room to draw, the children refused to draw until the black colors had been returned. It was hypothesized by the therapists that traumatized children preferred specific colors (in this case, black), and that through color use they were able to express their psychological pain to

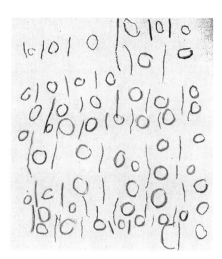

FIGURE 5.30. Drawing by a 4-year-old boy with repetitions of shape and lines. From "LA '94 Earthquake in eyes of children: Art Therapy with Elementary School Children Who Were Victims of Disaster" by Jasenka Roje, in Art Therapy: Journal of the American Art Therapy Association, 12(4), 237–243. Copyright 1995 by the American Art Therapy Association, Inc. All rights reserved. Reprinted by permission.

the world: anxiety, helplessness, loneliness, sadness, feeling threatened, vulnerable, fearfulness, even terror and despair.

The therapists who worked with the child survivors observed another unusual use of black in the children's art expressions: the appearance of a black sun (Figures 5.32 and 5.33). The image of a black sun has been related to darkness, death, fear, terror, melancholy, and desperation (Gregorian et al., 1996), although none of the young children who were part of the study described their images with similar meaning. However, given the devastating effects of the catastrophe they had experienced, it is apparent that severe depression, fear, anxiety, and symptoms of PTSD could be related to including such a potent image in their art expressions.

RESILIENCE AND TRAUMA

Children, like adults, react to traumatic circumstances differently. Some seem to react with great emotion, some become withdrawn, and others may be susceptible to the long-term effects of PTSD. Many children, however, may rebound or recover quickly, having a natural

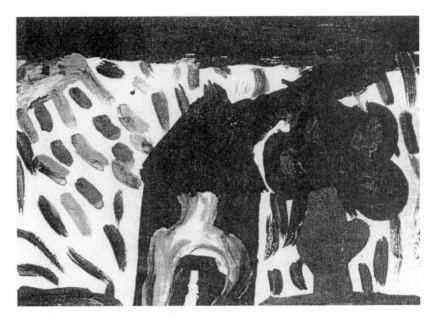

FIGURE 5.31. Child's drawing after the Armenian earthquake. From "Colors of Disaster: The Psychology of the 'Black Sun,'" by Vitali S. Gregorian, Anait Azarian, Michael DeMaria, and Leisl D. McDonald, in *The Arts in Psychotherapy, 23*(1), 1–14. Copyright 1996 by Elsevier Science Ltd. Reprinted by permission.

adaptability and resiliency in the face of circumstances that seriously debilitate others. Others, although depressed or fearful, display coping skills and personality traits that demonstrate their propensity to improve and recover. Often, in looking for signs of disturbance, difficulties, and problems, therapists overlook the possibility of children's drawings expressing their strengths, skills, and abilities to deal with and overcome traumatic events.

Resiliency is a term that refers to the ability to recover from depression, adversity, illness, or other negative situations. For children, resiliency is defined as the "capacity of those who are exposed to identifiable risk factors to overcome those risks and avoid negative outcomes such as delinquency and behavioral problems, psychological maladjustment, academic difficulties, and physical complications" (Rak & Patterson, 1996, p. 368). Children who are resilient have an ability to maintain a positive and meaningful view of life, are able to actively problem solve, have a sense of optimism, are proactive, and seek out new experiences (Werner, 1992). Of course, resiliency may be predicated upon many things, including social support from family

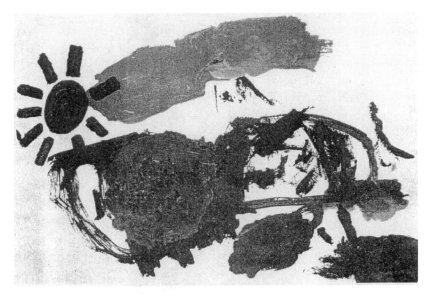

FIGURE 5.32. Drawing with black sun by child after the Armenian earthquake. From "Colors of Disaster: The Psychology of the'Black Sun,'" by Vitali S. Gregorian, Anait Azarian, Michael DeMaria, and Leisl D. McDonald, in *The Arts in Psychotherapy, 23*(1), 1–14. Copyright 1996 by Elsevier Science Ltd. Reprinted by permission.

and friends, nurturance in the first few years of life, and identified role models such as teachers, coaches, and therapists, but it is a quality that is often underestimated in children, particularly those who have grown up in difficult or traumatizing circumstances.

Unfortunately, not much is known about what drawings say about positive qualities such as resiliency and adaptability in children. Most studies of the emotional content of children's drawings have focused on potential problems rather than children's potentials to thrive. My own clinical experiences with children who exhibit resilience suggest to me that there may be some characteristics in their art expressions that are indicative of their resiliency. Many of these characteristics are not easily quantifiable, but nevertheless they seem to underscore these children's positive self-regard for themselves and others, their enthusiasm for life, and hopeful views of the future. For example, many children who have been abused or come from abusive or violent homes, despite their experiences, display and describe positive aspects in their drawings, ones that emphasize their abilities to cope effectively with trauma and to find meaning and hope in the world around them. For example,

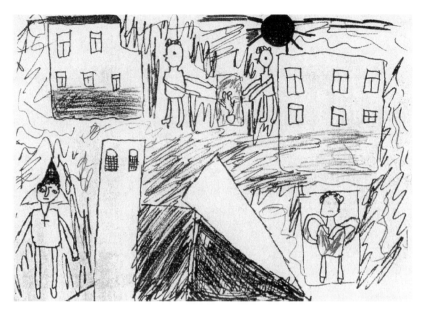

FIGURE 5.33. Drawing with black sun by child after the Armenian earthquake. From "Colors of Disaster: The Psychology of the 'Black Sun,'" by Vitali S. Gregorian, Anait Azarian, Michael DeMaria, and Leisl D. McDonald, in *The Arts in Psychotherapy, 23*(1), 1–14. Copyright 1996 by Elsevier Science Ltd. Reprinted by permission.

a 7-year-old boy from an abusive home, when asked to draw a self-portrait (Figure 5.34), drew a large image of himself with a broad smile, noting that "things are pretty bad with my family right now, but they are going to get better someday for me and my sister." This sense of hopefulness, both in his confident self-image and his verbal description, is key to resiliency and indicates a belief in an internal, rather than external, sense of control of one's life. Other children from abusive or violent homes may express their resiliency through wishful images of a positive home life, such as Joanne's drawings of nurturing and stable family environments (Figure 5.16).

Some children may draw images that depict themselves as active, rather than passive, participants in life, indicating that they see themselves as having an effect on their own situations as well as those of others. Tibbetts (1989) notes in his work with children who lived through violence in Northern Ireland that some children in his study drew pictures that represented active attempts to resolve or overcome traumatic feelings. This sense of being able to influence events seems to be a type of resilience that certain children have, despite over-

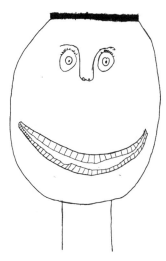

FIGURE 5.34. A 7-year-old boy's drawing of himself as happy and confident.

whelming circumstances, and their art may depict their active attempts to resolve their feelings and the circumstances that are troubling them.

Children's drawings preserved from the Nazi concentration camp
at Terezin, Czechoslovakia, are an important testament to the resiliency of children who were profoundly traumatized. Approximately
4,000 drawings were saved, and although many of the drawings in this
collection depict scenes and events connected to life in concentration
camps and the Holocaust, children also created images representing
things of beauty: distant or imagined landscapes, animals, birds and
butterflies, children playing, and memories of previous homes and
family life. Some of these images may have been assigned as subjects
or activities by teachers at the camp as part of art instruction; this
may, in part, account for some of their themes. However, for the most
part, the art expressions are not specifically focused on Nazi inhumanity and cruelty, but instead record both daily events and impressions
that convey hope and faith. The art expressions of these children
demonstrate their need to express themselves and their abilities to
make sense of profoundly tragic and horrific circumstances. As
Golomb (1990) notes, the drawings are "also an act of spiritual defi-
ance in the face of overwhelming powers amassed by the Nazis to de-
stroy any trace of their victims' existence" (p. 148).

These are but very few examples of how children's art expressions can provide therapists with windows to understanding more positive personality and emotional qualities such as positive self-regard, optimism, hope, and adaptability. Although therapists who use drawings with children to understand what possibly might represent negative, painful, or worrisome emotions should also realize that the realm of art expression also includes the other end of the spectrum. There are fortunately many children, for whom, despite painful personal experiences and distressing family lives, art seems to be a place of joy and hope in contrast to the loss, anger, anxiety, or fears they may be experiencing. These children are not necessarily in denial or defended about their traumas, fears, or sadness; they simply find drawing to be a positive way to communicate and an activity that allows them to create positive world views or to imagine other possibilities and scenarios. Drawing and art making are undoubtedly experiences that can contain unspeakable pain and troublesome feelings, but they are also activities that bring pleasure and a measure of safety and can reveal children's potentials to adapt, cope, and thrive in what may seem to be overwhelming circumstances. This aspect of art expression may, in and of itself, be conducive to supporting resiliency in children, a far more important aspect than merely regarding drawings as simple reflections of emotional states.

CONCLUSION

Although children struggling with painful feelings, trauma, or crisis often express their feelings through art, it is important to realize that emotional content takes on many forms and is affected by many factors, including developmental influences and the context. Therapists are often in the business of looking for problems, signs of emotional difficulty, or the effects of stress in the children they see. While this is an important part of work with traumatized or emotionally distressed children, it seems equally logical that a possibility exists for seeing potentials in children through their art, particularly emotional strengths that can be reinforced in therapy to serve these children outside of the session. A focus on emotional health can help mental health professionals who work with children to understand that children's needs to express themselves through creative activities such as drawing are not only images of trauma, crisis, or pain, but also are efforts toward finding health, well-being, and emotional wholeness.

Interpersonal Aspects
of Children's Drawings

The term "interpersonal" can be defined as interactions with another person or persons and is an expression often associated with group dynamics and family work. Interpersonal relationships are especially emphasized in the field of family therapy, where people and events are viewed in the context of connection and mutual influence. Rather than regarding people as separate from others and their environment, this perspective seeks to understand people as responding to a larger system including families, extended families, significant others, communities, and society.

Children are greatly influenced by interpersonal relationships with their parents, siblings, relatives, friends, and teachers (and therapists) and reflect their impressions of these interactions in their art expressions. Children's images of neighborhoods, school, and communities can be considered reflections of themselves, but they also are images of what children see, feel, experience, and think about other people and the environment. Although interpersonal aspects of children's drawings could be addressed as part of the emotional content of their creative work, these aspects also reflect children's views of self in relation to others and really deserve consideration from an interpersonal perspective.

In this chapter, three types of drawings that often reflect children's interpersonal views are described: children's drawings of their families and what can be understood from family drawings; children's drawings of houses with an emphasis on how these drawings may be useful in understanding interpersonal dynamics and children's perceptions of home, environment, and community; and children's drawings of the therapist, which are useful in understanding how the child relates to and perceives a helping adult. A short discussion of gender and children's drawings is also included, since gender is a characteristic that not only reflects self-perception but also reflects how children see themselves in relation to others.

CHILDREN'S DRAWINGS OF THEIR FAMILIES

Family drawings are a logical place to begin when considering how children express their interpersonal views. Many mental health professionals who use drawing with children believe children's family drawings communicate information on family dynamics through content, placement, size of figures, as well as the process of constructing the drawing (Burns & Kaufman, 1972; Burns, 1982; Oster & Gould, 1987; Oster & Montgomery, 1996). Drawings of families are popular assignments in therapeutic work with children, since understanding family interactions is generally an important issue in treatment.

Family drawings frequently have been used as a part of assessment as well as a method of therapeutic communication in work with children. Professionals who work with children often ask them to draw their families, usually as part of an evaluation or as a means of gathering additional information about their perceptions of family life. Social workers and protective service personnel regularly request a family drawing from children whose families are having problems or are suspected of domestic violence or child abuse. As a part of an overall assessment, children's drawings of their families are thought to enhance therapists' understanding of not only children's feelings about themselves but also how they perceive themselves in relation to people who are significant in their lives and how they view systems, hierarchies, and boundaries within their families. For these reasons, children's drawings of their families may be helpful in identifying the need for further intervention in the form of family counseling.

Using family drawings as part of assessment with children is not a new idea and was employed as early as the 1930s as a projective drawing task. Appel (1931) and Wolff (1942) first suggested that children's drawings of their families might provide insight into personality. Later, Hulse (1952) collected and studied numerous children's drawings of their families, comparing both normal children's drawings and those of children who were considered emotionally disturbed. Hulse's studies focused on understanding the total appearance of children's family drawings, rather than singular characteristics. He observed that children project both deep emotional feelings about parents and siblings and family dynamics within the home situation in their family drawings.

Recently, a great deal of emphasis and meaning has been placed on specific signs and symbols found within children's family drawings. Although many therapists simply ask children to "draw your family," others use the Kinetic Family Drawing (KFD; Burns & Kaufman, 1972), a widely employed drawing task. The procedure asks the child to "draw a picture of everyone in your family, including you, doing something. Try to draw whole people, not cartoons or stick people. Remember, make everyone doing something—some kind of action" (Burns & Kaufman, 1972, p. 5). The part about "doing something" within the directive is emphasized in order encourage children to draw images that include action between the figures. As with other projective drawing tasks, it is thought that children can express ideas, feelings, and perceptions through family drawings more easily than through words.

In addition to understanding family dynamics from the child's point of view, the KFD task is thought to be a visual record of self-development within a family system, especially if drawings are collected over time. However, like many projective drawing tasks, the KFD has been criticized by those who question the validity of interpreting characteristics, signs, and symbols in children's drawings of their families (Golomb, 1990). Although a great deal of attention has been given to family drawings, it is difficult to say how much they really reveal about family dynamics and what particular characteristics are significant. The body of research produced on children's depictions of their families, including data on the KFD, is minimal, and what has been observed has not been replicated on a large scale.

While therapists may be inclined to interpret the content and style of children's drawings of their families, it is important to be judicious in one's interpretation and to consider all the aspects mentioned throughout this book in making any judgments. Because family drawings involve a series of human figures, a great deal of speculation has resulted on why children position family members in relation to each other in various ways or draw visual boundaries (the use of lines to separate, compartmentalize, or encapsulate figures) between figures. Although how children position figures and visual boundaries may provide some clues to their perceptions of family relationships, it is pretty difficult to say with any degree of certainty what exactly these characteristics mean for individual children. For example, while encapsulation or separation of figures from one another within a drawing is thought to be a form of avoidance of others (Burns & Kaufman, 1972), with some children and in certain situations, this characteristic could be understood as an expression of seeking safety or even independence. In families where inappropriate or even abusive behaviors are occuring (such as physical maltreatment or sexual abuse), a child may try symbolically to establish boundaries within a drawing as an adaptive coping skill as a means of protection or escape. In other cases, it may be a result of simply wanting or needing to have one's own "space." Children have their own unique reasons for positioning figures in specific ways. Because there are a variety of possible meanings, therapists will want to talk with children about their family drawings in order to get more information.

When requesting family drawings from children, it is also important to consider that drawing a family is not usually a favorite subject of children when given freedom to draw anything they want. Unlike other drawings children do, most family drawings in my experience are not spontaneous; that is, when given the opportunity to draw anything they want, children do not seem to draw families. The exception seems to be children in Stage III (ages 4 to 6 years), a time when human figures become an important part of drawings, and children naturally draw images of themselves, their parents, siblings, and other people who are significant to them. School-aged children (such as those in Stages IV and V, 6 years and older) do not seem to make impromptu drawings of their families, and in order to get a drawing of a family from a child, the therapist usually has to specifically request one.

When asked to simply "draw a picture of your family," children who are well-adjusted and comfortable with their families generally draw images that are often charming and creative, capturing details of family life and remarkably unique characteristics of parents, siblings, and self. Seven-year-old Ian's drawing of his family (Figure 6.1) shows himself as the youngest family member, his older sister Emily, mother Lori, father Fred, and the family dog, Ruby. Ian is very careful about details such as clothing and color (including hair color) in his drawings and likes to include details, such as an overhead light. For his age, Ian's drawing is fairly sophisticated, and he is able to draw figures with not only great detail and precision but also has accurately represented

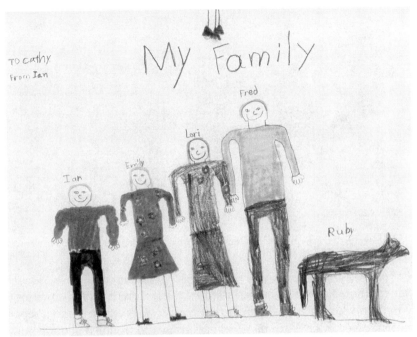

FIGURE 6.1. Seven-year-old Ian's drawing of his family.

the members of his family in terms of relative size and individual features. I particularly enjoy his personal treatment of feet which he usually draws facing in the same direction (see Figure 4.20 of a baseball player and Batman, and Figure 6.17 later in this chapter).

In contrast to children who are well-adjusted, children who are under a great deal of stress or are concerned about family problems, may find making a family drawing difficult or even anxiety producing. Children may be hesitant for reasons of safety or because they have negative feelings about family life or are fearful of repercussions for portraying a family secret. Drawing people, especially families, seems to bring up issues, both positive and negative, in children's lives. In my work with children who are traumatized by family violence, the question "draw your family doing something" usually yields mixed results. Sometimes children do draw their family members engaged in an activity, but more often they draw a series of figures lined up in a row (Figure 6.2). Despite the request to draw their families in action, this child population either resists or is unable to draw them at all.

Other children do not want to draw their families because they

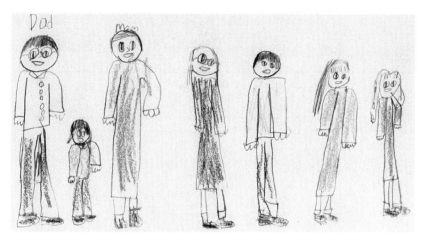

FIGURE 6.2. Drawing of a "family doing something" showing figures lined up in a row.

are conflicted about or embarrassed by their current family situation. Children who are from a family that has recently experienced a separation, divorce, or death may feel uncertain and troubled about whom to include in their family picture. Although it has been noted that noncompliance is rare among children who are asked to draw their families doing something, when children are afraid or confused about their family situation, they may decline or ignore the request. Asking these children to draw their family may be too threatening, especially if requested early in the therapeutic relationship and before a good deal of trust has been established. Hulse (1952) noted that family drawings done by children at school were much more elaborate and detailed than those done in the therapist's office or clinic, underscoring that a visit to a clinician may provoke anxiety, suspicion, and resistance in many children.

Additionally, drawing one's family is a complicated task, and in some situations, overwhelming. For example, where I live, families are often quite large due to the predominant religion (the Latter Day Saints, which encourages large families), and children in therapy can be frustrated with the task of drawing 8, 10, or 12 people (plus the family pets, who are frequently included in their family pictures). It is difficult to draw a great many people, and in many cases, children, including those who normally draw realistically, tend to hastily draw a set of stick figures (Figure 6.3) to represent their numerous family members. When so many figures are included in a single drawing,

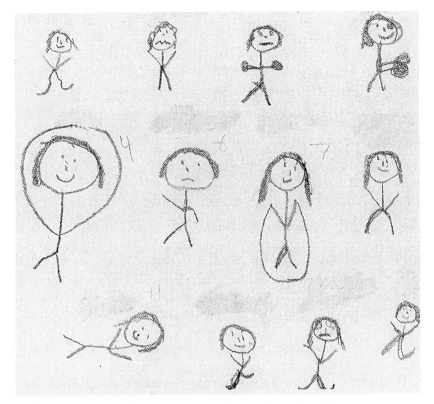

FIGURE 6.3. An 11-year-old's family drawing comprised of stick figures to represent numerous family members.

many children understandably find it hard to accurately plan where the figures will be placed, sometimes even running out of space on the standard 8½″ × 11″ paper. When a child approaches a family drawing in this way, it is hard to say what the image means in terms of relative size or placement of figures except that drawing one's large family is an exhausting task.

The stage of artistic development also has an impact on children's drawings of their families. For example, in Stage III when children first draw prototypes for people and early human figures, placement is difficult to judge because children at this stage freely place images throughout the composition. Children in the stage of realism (Stage V) are sometimes reluctant to draw their families because they are not able to make the drawing appear photographically correct. On occasion a preadolescent or adolescent will regress to an earlier form of expression such as stick figures in order to comply with the assignment (such as in Figure 6.3). It is very difficult to draw one's family at any age and when asked to draw one's family engaged in activities, it is a complex task that even adults will resist. Family drawings are exercises that therapists themselves should attempt in order to fully understand the degree of difficulty this directive entails. Taking time to draw one's own family will give the therapist a good sense of the complexity and frustration that come with this activity.

DRAWINGS OF FAMILY MEMBERS

As an alternative to asking children to draw a complete family picture or image of an entire family doing something, I frequently ask children to draw themselves with a family member of their own choosing, in an effort to alleviate some of the stress they may experience with drawing their entire family. Children's drawings of specific family members can be surprisingly revealing, and this seems to be a less threatening introduction to drawing the family because it gives children control in choosing whom to depict. It allows children the opportunity to focus on their most significant other(s) and to identify family support(s) both to themselves and to the therapist. It also provides a format for expressing feelings of concern or loss about separation from a significant person in their lives. For example, when asked to draw himself with a family member, a 6-year-old boy at a shelter for battered women drew himself with his father (Figure 6.4). The drawing quickly brought out the anxieties the boy had about an upcoming divorce hearing in which custody of the children would be decided. The child was fearful that he would have to go with his mother and would never see his father again. The drawing of the father was relevant not only because it provided a way to express feelings about his parent, but it also reduced some anxieties the boy was having about separation.

Figure 6.5, a pencil drawing by a 5-year-old physically abused boy, shows his grandmother and himself. In talking with the therapist about the drawing, he described his grandmother as a positive and reliable social support in his life. Although the boy lived with his mother, she was not the person he chose to draw, possibly because she was often emotionally unavailable and was not effective in stopping the abuse. In contrast, the grandmother was often the boy's caretaker and protected him from several incidents of physical abuse and punish-

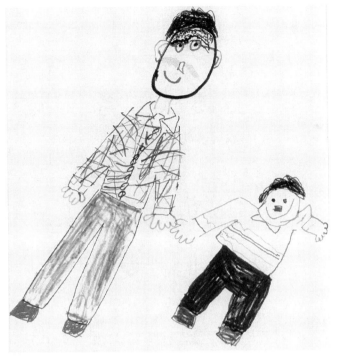

FIGURE 6.4. A 6-year-old boy's drawing of himself and his father.

ment. Although the boy was not comfortable with drawing any other members of his family, he spontaneously volunteered to the therapist while completing the drawing that his father was a bad man who had a gun and later that his mother hit him sometimes, confirming that she had indeed been abusive.

A therapist interested in children's views of family may also ask children to draw their "favorite" people. Figure 6.6 shows a 7-year-old girl's drawing of favorite people, within an exercise to also draw favorite foods, places, and things to do, and things that scare her. She identified her mother, grandmother and new baby brother as three favorite people, leaving out her father who was abusive to her and her mother. The directive to draw "things that scare me" gave her the opportunity to include her father as one of two monsters in that section. This example underscores the importance of allowing children who are fearful or anxious about particular family members a way to express these emotions without feeling pressured to include them within a family portrait.

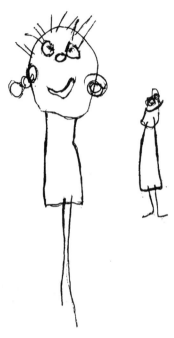

FIGURE 6.5. A 6-year-old boy's drawing of himself and his grandmother. From *Breaking the Silence* by Cathy A. Malchiodi. Copyright 1997 by Brunner/Mazel. Reprinted by permission.

Gillespie (1994, 1997) has explored the use of mother-and-child drawings in her work with projective assessments. The directive asks the child to "draw a mother and child," in order to encourage a drawing that may indicate how the child sees relationships, particularly the primary one between mother and child. Although the task does not specifically request that the child draw his or her own mother, it is thought to be a useful way to understand issues of early development from an object relations perspective, emphasizing delays, symbiosis, merger, separation, and individuation (Gillespie, 1997). Although the task does not seem to be reliable in identifying specific disorders in children, it may be a helpful addition to understanding how children relate to parents or primary caretakers.

Lastly, drawings of family members also can be a useful way to help mental health professionals and others who work with children to understand their social values and world views. Children view parents, siblings, and other relatives through their own special lenses; through drawing significant individuals in their lives, they can convey

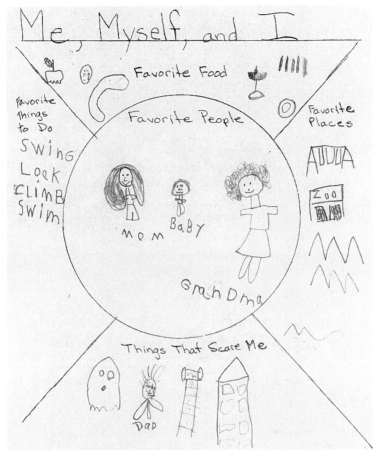

FIGURE 6.6. Drawing of "favorite family members" by a 7-year-old girl.

personal perceptions and communicate beliefs and attitudes about them. For example, in a small study of children's drawings of elderly individuals, children expressed their perceptions of old age through narratives and art expression (Weber, Cooper, & Hesser, 1996). The children, ages 8 to 11 years, were asked to "draw a picture of an old person" and to talk about the characteristics and features of their drawings. Since most children learned about older people through grandparents, their drawings reflected what they perceived about these older family members. While the children's narratives about their pictures provided important information about their views of old age, their images were equally revealing. For example, a 9-year-old girl depicted a 99-year-old woman dancing (Figure 6.7), a picture of her grandmother who, she said, liked to dance and who the girl hoped to teach how to use a skateboard. Although the image may reflect the girl's own interests in rock and roll music and dance, it does convey her perceptions of her grandparent as being vigorous and active. Most of the children in the study did not see old age as a negative experience and often depicted elderly people as happy, energetic, and active in their drawings.

Undoubtedly, drawings of the self and family members provide children a way to communicate interpersonal perspectives not easily expressed through other types of drawings. With appropriate use and careful consideration of the child, family drawings can be helpful in understanding children's feelings about family life, particularly in areas of connectedness and social support. Although not addressed in this brief section, family drawings also have the potential to reveal changes in children's perceptions of belonging in their families over

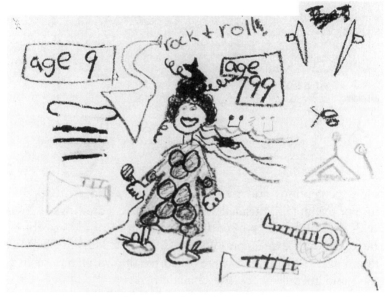

FIGURE 6.7. Drawing of her 99-year-old grandmother "dancing" by a 9-year-old girl. From "Children's Drawings of the Elderly: Young Ideas Abandon Old Age Stereotypes" by Joseph Weber, Kathy Cooper, and Jenny Hesser, in *Art Therapy: Journal of the American Art Therapy Association*, 13(2), 114–117. Copyright 1996 by the American Art Therapy Association, Inc. All rights reserved. Reprinted by permission.

time (Burns, 1982) and improvement in family relationships as a result of therapy or changes in communication patterns between family members. If a therapist has the luxury of seeing a child over a long period of time, family drawings and drawings of family members can be helpful in noting children's changing perceptions of their primary relationships with parents, guardians, and significant others.

HOUSE DRAWINGS AND
INTERPERSONAL PERSPECTIVES

Children's drawings of houses have usually been considered from an intrapsychic perspective rather than an interpersonal one, with an emphasis on how they reflect individual personality. Much has been written about the psychological importance of house drawings, including characteristics that have been associated with personality traits or mental disturbance (Buck, 1948). There has also been a great deal of emphasis on individual features, such as the inclusion of doors, windows, and chimneys with or without smoke, and connections have been made between these characteristics and personality, intelligence, neurological problems, or emotional disturbance.

In trying to understand children's perceptions of their homes and family life, many therapists do naturally wonder about certain characteristics in children's house drawings, particularly chimneys, chimney smoke, and floating houses. These characteristics have been noted throughout the literature on projective drawings and have been related to both self-perception and to interpersonal aspects (Buck, 1948; Jolles, 1971). Although I do not believe in unilaterally subscribing any particular meaning to singular characteristics in children's drawings, I have to admit that these specific characteristics have fascinated me also, particularly because children recreate these elements in intriguing ways.

Chimneys on house drawings seem to consistently generate the most questions and attention from therapists, have been assigned conflicting meanings, and, as a result, their implications in children's drawings are confusing. Chimneys have been associated with interpersonal warmth between family members and, on the other hand, given phallic significance by some (Jolles, 1971). Smoke coming out the chimney also seems to capture many people's imaginations, and therapists often wonder or make note of children's inclusion of smoke (especially profuse smoke) coming from chimneys on children's house drawings. Chimney smoke has been related to anger or inner tension within the individual or, on an interpersonal level, within the household between people (Oster & Gould, 1987), but the data are not very convincing given the fact that so many children regularly include smoke coming out of chimneys on house drawings. In my experience it is hard to say what, if any significance, smoke coming out of chimney has or if there is some important or hidden meaning to its inclusion. Nevertheless, chimney smoke regularly appears in children's drawings, particularly those in Stage IV, when schemata become important in artistic expression (Figure 6.8).

Floating houses, defined as houses that are not resting on a baseline or edge of the paper, also appear in children's drawings of houses and environments. Very young children will commonly draw houses without concern for placement or groundlines. Therefore, it is not unusual to see an ungrounded house or an upside-down house for that matter, in their drawings. In Stage IV where visual schemata are important, a groundline is included or the edge of the paper is used for the base on which to draw a house. However, other children, when asked to draw a house, pragmatically draw what is asked of them and do not include a baseline; this seems to be particularly true when they are only

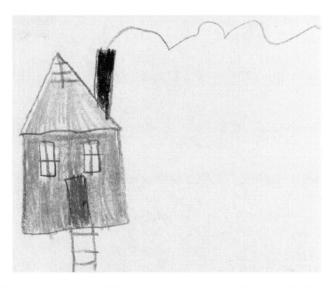

FIGURE 6.8. Six-year-old children's house drawings with chimney smoke. (continued on next page)

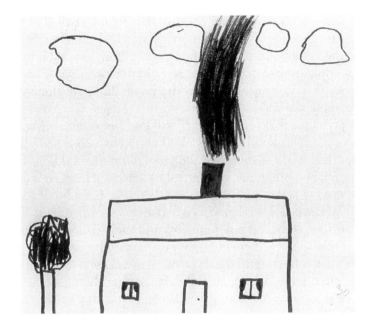

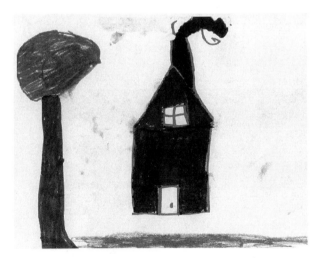

FIGURE 6.8 (continued from previous page)

given a lead pencil rather than colored drawing materials that might stimulate the drawing of grass or ground. When I ask children why they didn't draw a groundline for their house, they often respond by saying, "Well, you asked me to draw a house, so I just drew a house." Therefore, what looks like a floating house without a groundline may simply be the child's compliance with the directive of the therapist.

In my clinical experience with children from violent homes or transitory lifestyles and homeless children, I have seen many house drawings that are floating above the groundline the child has drawn (Figure 6.9), and others are surrounded by a maze of lines, as if caught up in a tornado or wind storm (Figure 6.10). It is difficult not to speculate about the possible connections between these ungrounded houses and at times turbulent environments and these children's inconsistent and often violent home life. However, it is also important to remember that a floating house drawing may, in some cases, indicate that the child has a developmental delay or that there is some other influence at work. When seeing a house that is floating or ungrounded drawn by a child who should be in Stage IV or older, the therapist may consider the possibility of developmental delays, particularly if the child is also having problems in school with learning disabilities.

Although actual details of house drawings such as chimneys, windows, doors, and other details are interesting, stories children tell

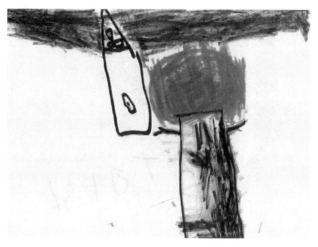

FIGURE 6.9. House floating above a groundline by a 6-year-old boy from a violent home.

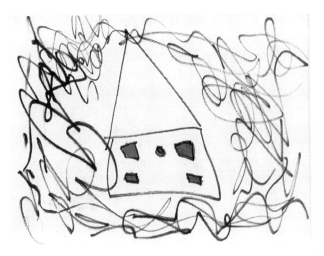

FIGURE 6.10. House floating amid a maze of lines by a 7-year-old girl from a violent home.

about house drawings are usually much more informative and can tell the therapist more about family life within the home than can singular characteristics. House drawings are really environmental drawings, so there is an opportunity not only to ask about the features of the house itself but also about what is going on inside and outside of the house. In this sense, drawings of houses are an effective way to understand children's interpersonal relationships. Houses embody children's impressions of family life and other significant relationships and ideas about their relationship to the environment. They naturally invite stories not only about who lives in them and what goes on inside them, but also the neighborhood and environment where the house is located. There are a number of ways the therapist can go about this (see Chapter 3 for more information on working with drawings) and children seem to enjoy providing stories about their house images.

Houses may also reveal slightly different information about who lives with the family than a standard family drawing. For example, a child may not include a family friend or divorced mother's boyfriend in a family drawing but, when asked about who lives in their house, may communicate that information. Additionally, children are usually amenable to drawing houses, finding them less frustrating to draw than human figures, and are generally more comfortable talking about them.

Sometimes I ask children for drawings of their homes when I sus-
pect that something is going on inside the home that may be important to know more about and especially if there is something going on
within the family that may be harmful to the child. In order to find
out even more specific information, I may ask the child to draw a particular house, such as "draw your house just before you go to school" or
"draw your house on Sunday morning." This prompts children to draw
a specific scene from their family life along with the house itself; it often results in X-ray drawings depicting what is going on inside the
home. For example, when asked to make a "drawing of your home at
night" (Figure 6.11), a 7-year-old girl drew everyone in bed: her two
sisters, brother, father and mother upstairs in their beds, and herself
downstairs in bed by the television. When I asked her about the sleep-
ing arrangements, particularly why she slept away from the family in a
downstairs bed, she said that it was "so my dad can come down to my
bed at night and jump on me." The girl was being sexually abused by
her father during the night and was kept separate from the rest of the
family in order to accommodate him. The drawing provides some other important details; for example, the television, drawn as the largest
object in the picture, apparently was turned on during the abuse in order to muffle the sounds of the girl being abused.

Asking children about who lives in their neighborhood (or
apartment or condominium complex) when talking with them about
their house drawings can also provide some important information.
Often children will talk about friends whom they play with (or have
fights with) and other individuals outside the family who live in the
immediate vicinity. When I am wondering from a therapeutic standpoint about the amount and quality of social support a child has outside the family, this can be useful. Some children will also volunteer
information about conflicts within their neighborhood, and this is often helpful in understanding their world views. For example, when
asked to draw a picture of his house, an 8-year-old boy drew the duplex (i.e., two-family home) where he lived with his mother and sister
(Figure 6.12). He described the home as "big and I have my own
room," but when asked about the neighbors who lived in the other
part of the duplex, he said, "They're Mormons and we're Catholics, so
they don't let their children play with us. They have parties over there
all the time, but Mormons don't ask Catholics to come their parties."
Whether or not the degree of prejudice described by the child was
valid is difficult to determine; however, what is obvious is his belief

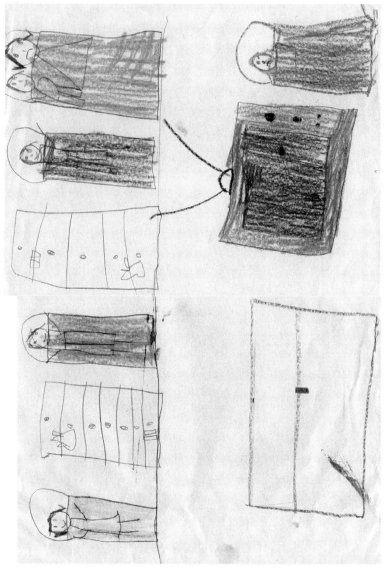

FIGURE 6.11. Drawing of home at night by a 7-year-old girl.

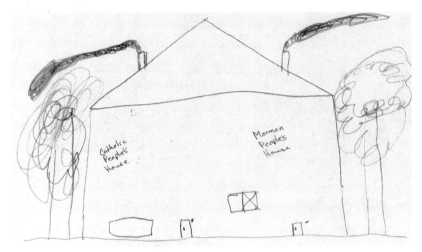

FIGURE 6.12. Drawing of two-family home by an 8-year-old boy.

that a conflict existed between his family and the family next door because of their religious differences.

In terms of what goes on inside a house, unless a child draws an X-ray or cut-away view of a house, the characteristics of a house drawing often do not provide much solid information about family life. When asked to draw a house, normally children draw minimal features such as a door and perhaps a few windows, a roof, chimney and occasionally a path leading up to the door. Again, asking some simple questions about the drawing yield more information than the details of the drawing itself. Ten-year-old Rich's drawing of his house (Figure 6.13) emphasized his room but, when asked about who lives there, he stated that he lived there "with his mom, sister, and big brother, but not his stepdad because he is too mean. Our real dad that lives in New Jersey can come and stay with us any time." This single drawing and Rich's description provided the therapist with a quick portrait of who was living in the home and additional information on their relationship with the biological father who lived outside the state. An 8-year-old girl's minimal drawing of a house shaped like a tee-pee (Figure 6.14) provided very few details, but her verbal description of the rooms inside the house clarified that her mother and father slept in separate beds upstairs, an important piece for the therapist in understanding the family dynamics.

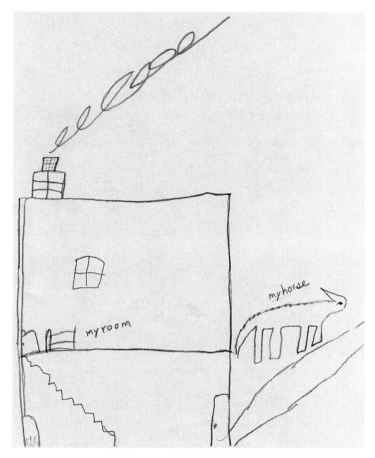

FIGURE 6.13. A 10-year-old boy's drawing of home.

INTERPERSONAL RELATIONSHIP
WITH THE THERAPIST

Several chapters in this book have touched on the importance of the therapist's relationship with children and its influence on their images. In that same vein, drawings of the therapist can provide another window to the therapeutic alliance and are another source of how children perceive and represent significant relationships in their lives. These images often appear spontaneously during the course of therapy, although they can be requested if one is brave enough to withstand seeing the results! Children will usually present an interesting portrait of the therapist or, at the very least, surprising features, often empha-

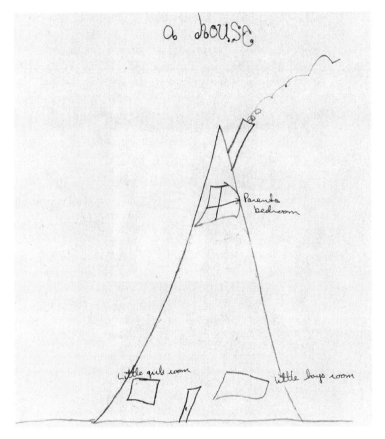

a house

Parents bedroom

little girls room   little boys room

FIGURE 6.14. An 8-year-old girl's drawing of home shaped like a tee-pee.

sizing the aspects that are the most prominent to them. My glasses, for example, always seem to play a large part in children's portraits of me, perhaps since at times they have been large or unusual (according to the current fashion) or perhaps because I am almost always intent on watching what children are drawing or creating during a session (Figure 6.15).

Children can also be quite observant of various characteristics and behaviors of the therapist that can clarify the child's perceptions about the therapist and treatment. For example, in Figure 6.16, a drawing by a girl at a battered women's shelter visually describes some important characteristics such as large ears, which were for listening (this therapist's native language was not English, and she had to listen carefully in order to understand American speech) and prominent

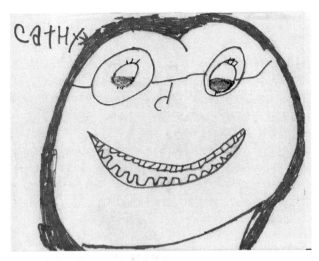

FIGURE 6.15. Drawing of the therapist by a child. From *Breaking the Silence* by Cathy A. Malchiodi. Copyright 1997 by Brunner/Mazel. Reprinted by permission.

eyes for watching what she was drawing. This girl was keenly aware that the therapist was extremely interested in what she was saying and doing, perhaps almost to the point of suspicion. The girl also wrote "art teacher" on her paper, revealing some confusion about what a therapist is, particularly a therapist who uses drawings with children. In many environments, such as shelters, hospitals, or clinics, the child may be confused about who the therapist is and why he or she is there to help; drawings may make visible perceptions of the helping adult that a child may be hesitant to say or cannot articulate in words. This information is valuable feedback to the therapist in understanding from a child's perspective how he or she sees the therapist and therapy and in determining the need for further clarification of the helping relationship.

According to Rubin (1984a), children may view a therapist in a variety of ways: nurturing, permissive, restrictive, demanding, probing, or mean, among other things. The therapist may be represented as one or a combination of these perceptions and, at times, in an unflattering manner. The therapist must understand that these perceptions may mean many things and can involve transference issues specific to the child's experiences of adults in general, parents, or caretakers. For example, with children who have been traumatized by violence in the home or physically or sexually abused, their drawings of

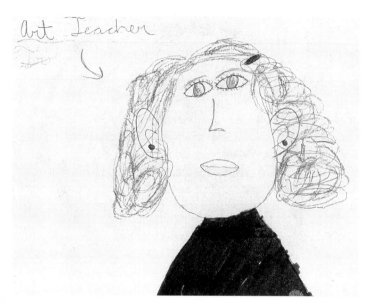

FIGURE 6.16. Drawing of the therapist by a child. From *Breaking the Silence* by Cathy A. Malchiodi. Copyright 1997 by Brunner/Mazel. Reprinted by permission.

the therapist may be indicative of their feelings about adult figures in general: The therapist may be portrayed as controlling, punishing, unreliable, abusive, or unstable, despite the therapist's best efforts to the contrary. The therapist may be also represented as powerful and omnipotent, and the child may have fantasies that the therapist can transform an unhappy family situation or reunite separated parents. The child may have unrealistic hopes involving rescue and nurturance when the therapist is perceived this way, conveying excessive dependence, a maladaptive coping pattern common to crisis.

GENDER AND CHILDREN'S DRAWINGS

Although there are many aspects of children's drawings that touch on interpersonal issues, the role of gender is certainly one area that is important for therapists in understanding children's drawings. Unfortunately, while many therapists may wonder about how gender affects children's drawings, there is very little specific research on this topic, and the influence of gender in children's drawings remains perplexing.

Society and culture certainly shape what boys and girls draw, and children's art expressions are formed, to some extent, by traditional gender roles and images of gender in the media and literature and impacted by the gender values and beliefs of adults with whom children come in contact.

The topic of gender and children's drawings could have easily fit into other chapters of this book, particularly developmental aspects. A few studies of children's art expressions have explored the connections between gender and artistic development, although relatively little attention has been given to this topic in terms of formal studies. Gardner (1982), in his extensive work with children and artistic activity, concludes that there may be some gender differences in how very young children express themselves through art. He observes that girls tend to sing during art making or employ expressive voices, and they excel in mixed media and combine gestures, symbolic play, narrations, and three-dimensional forms. Boys, according to Gardner's research, are more likely to excel with clay or single-medium tasks; often, they have a perpetual fascination with a certain character or superhero such as Batman. Batman has been a long-time favorite subject of Ian who drew the picture of his family shown earlier in this chapter (Figure 6.17) and he does seem to turn up frequently in drawings made by young boys.

With regard to artistic development, gender characteristics in human figure drawings are first visible at age 6, usually in the form of clothing (e.g., dresses for girls and women, pants for boys and men), although on occasion I have seen younger children who include simple details that differentiate boys and girls. During the schematic stage (Stage IV, 6 to 9 years), children not only begin to include recognizable schematic representations for clothing but also hairstyle that distinguishes boys and girls. In later stages, this interest in differentiating genders is apparent in preadolescent and adolescent drawings, and exploration of the gender differences through portraiture (Figure 6.18) is strongly evident.

Levick (1997), from her many years of experience in working with children, makes an interesting anecdotal observation about the appearance of gender differentiation in children's drawings:

> When I first began practicing art therapy in the 1960s, while television was still enjoying its innocence, I learned that most children draw stick figures at about age 7. This was expected behavior, because children

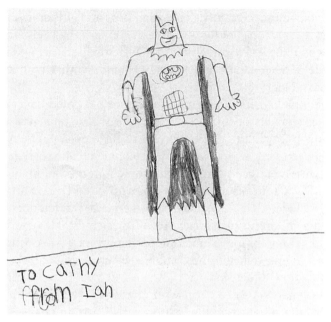

FIGURE 6.17. "Batman" by Ian.

usually are interested in differentiating between the sexes. . . . In the 1970s, changes in the stick figures became noticeable. Children between ages 7 and 9 were beginning to draw sexual characteristics on their figures, differentiating between male and female . . . it was becoming natural for children to draw sexual characteristics at an earlier age than in the past because children were seeing an emphasis on female/male characteristics/differences on television. (pp. 9–10)

Levick's observation underscores an important point about what may influence how children portray people and how these influences, such as television, videos, and more recently, the Internet, may affect the sexual content of children's drawings. These influences are becoming more apparent and have changed what were previously considered "norms" in the appearance of gender differentiation in children's art expressions.

Themes of children's drawings may also be gender-related. Golomb (1990) notes general differences in the themes of boys' and girls' drawings, observing that "the spontaneous productions of boys reveal an intense concern with warfare, acts of violence and destruc-

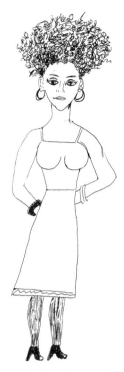

FIGURE 6.18. Drawing of a woman by an adolescent boy.

tion, machinery, and sports contests, whereas girls depict more tranquil scenes of romance, family life, landscapes, and children at play" (p. 158). She also finds that girls use fairy tales images such as kings and queens and animals such as horses as the subjects of their drawings. Whether this tendency to portray specific subjects by boys and girls is developmental or the result of parental or societal influences or both is not discussed by Golomb. However, these are undeniably gender-related themes commonly portrayed by boys and girls, and most therapists would probably agree that children, particularly those in the schematic stage of development (Stage IV), when drawing is an important story-telling activity, create drawings containing the subjects and themes suggested by Golomb.

Silver (1992, 1993, 1996b, 1997) has extensively explored the role of gender in children's drawings using the Draw-A-Story (DAS) task described in previous chapters to investigate possible differences in style and content of children's images. Silver's studies underscore the importance of interpreting how children depict subjects, themes, and verbal narratives for understanding of the role of gender in children's drawings.

One basic question Silver investigated through the DAS task was whether or not boys and girls chose to draw subjects of the same gender (i.e., boys draw pictures about male subjects, girls draw female subjects) in their drawings. A recent study (Silver, 1997) using the DAS with individuals of all ages did support the idea that most children and adolescents draw subjects of the same gender; however, some children and adolescents in the study did depict subjects of the opposite gender and did so in a surprising way. Silver found that of the children and adolescents who drew images that included subjects of the opposite gender, a significant number of them portrayed these subjects in a negative manner, depicting the subject as menacing, ridiculous, or hapless. Figure 6.19 is one example from the study, a drawing by a boy who used three stimulus drawings from the DAS (a bride, a knife, and a dog) to create an image titled "The lady getting married to a dog

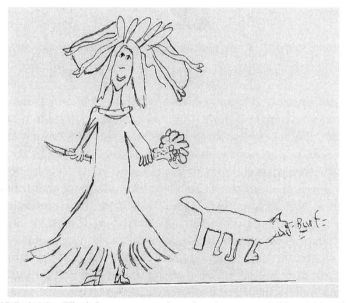

FIGURE 6.19. "The lady getting married to a dog who wants to kill him," Silver Drawing Test by an 8-year-old boy. From "Sex and Age Differences in Attitude toward the Opposite Sex" by Rawley Silver, in *Art Therapy: Journal of the American Art Therapy Association*, 14(4), 268–272. Copyright 1997 by the American Art Therapy Association, Inc. All rights reserved. Reprinted by permission.

who wants to kill him." Although the image could be considered humorous, it conveys a negative theme involving violence (e.g., the lady with a knife who wants to kill the dog). Children and adolescents of both genders drew and described the opposite gender in a negative manner; however, overall, male subjects were rated as more negative in the content of their drawings than female participants.

An earlier study (Silver, 1996b) looked at the DAS drawings of 138 adolescents, approximately half of whom were delinquent, wards of a juvenile court, and committed to a residential treatment facility; the other half were considered to be normal, attending schools where they lived. An interesting trend emerged in both group's drawings: More boys than girls drew pictures about assaultive relationships (i.e., an image depicting one subject acting violently or menacingly to another subject). However, in comparing the delinquent boys responses to those boys who were considered nondelinquent, more nondelinquent than delinquent boys in the study drew assaultive relationships. Silver hypothesized that this finding may be explained

> by the difference between fantasizing about violence and acting violently. A boy who has internalized prohibitions against acting out biological drives, may fantasize more than one who commits assaultive acts. It may also be that incarceration for antisocial behavior inhibited expressing assaultive fantasies." (pp. 548–549)

Some features that may be gender-related in children's and adolescent drawings are subtle in content and expression and may be representative of values, beliefs, and influences concerning gender of the society and culture where the individual lives. For example, in a small sample of self-portrait drawings (i.e., the adolescents were asked to draw a picture of themselves) collected from a classroom at a high school in the Midwest (Malchiodi, 1990), the influences of the dominant culture and its beliefs about gender roles are apparent. Within a group of 25 adolescent girls and 25 adolescent boys, two general themes emerged. The boys in the study always portrayed themselves as active and engaged in a sport or other action-oriented activity (Figure 6.20). The girls, in contrast, drew self-images that depicted either heads or full-body portraits (Figure 6.21), but none of the 25 drawings by the girls showed any type of movement or activity.

Since the local culture had strongly established rules based on the dominant religion for gender roles for males and females, these be-

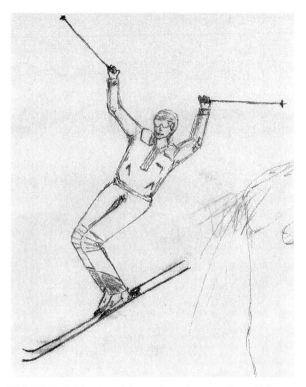

FIGURE 6.20. An adolescent boy's drawing of himself skiing.

liefs may have had a strong impact on these adolescent boys and girls and the content of their self-portraits. In this region, men are expected to be the heads of households, working outside the home, and leaders in the church, in other words, active in leadership roles and other activities. Women are encouraged to be homemakers, to have children, and to stay home if possible, a message that encourages a less active, more passive and traditional role for females. It seems likely that the content and themes of the adolescents in this particular sample may have been strongly influenced by the beliefs and values about gender roles in the community in which they were raised. However, if a more large-scale study of adolescent boys and girls drawings were conducted across the United States, similar features might also be found perhaps reflecting comparable beliefs systems and tendencies in gender roles.

The influence of gender on children's drawings is still a largely

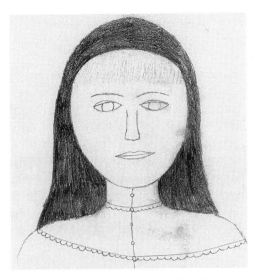

FIGURE 6.21. An adolescent girl's self-portait.

unexplored area, but it is still important to therapists in their under-standing of children's expressive work. It is obvious that children's perceptions of gender roles in society are often communicated to them by adults (parents, caretakers, teachers, and others) and influenced by what children see on television and movies, and read in books. There also may be some developmental aspects that influence how boys and girls create images that may be difficult to separate from societal and cultural influences but, nevertheless, that do exist. Although the overall understanding of the impact of gender in children's drawings is limited, therapists may learn a great deal not only about children's self-perceptions, but also their perceptions of those around them by considering gender's role in the style and content of art expressions.

CONCLUSION

Interpersonal aspects provide a different window for understanding children through their drawings. The uniquely narrative qualities of children's drawings of their families, homes, and home life offer im-portant information on how children see significant others in their lives. These drawings can be reflections of children's views of relation-ships, not only with parents, siblings, extended families, and friends but also how those relationships function within the larger community, whether it be within a neighborhood, school, or other environment.

Drawings have the ability not only to reflect children's unique personalities but also their unique perceptions and experiences with others as well as the influences of others. It is important to remember that drawings are not made in isolation from the world; parents, significant others, community, and society do affect the content of children's expressive work, and these interpersonal aspects are often included in their drawings. In this sense, children's drawings are uniquely individual narratives about themselves within the world, reflecting not only personality, but also personal observations, values, judgments, and perceptions of others and relationships to family, schools, community, and society.

CHAPTER SEVEN

Somatic and Spiritual Aspects of Children's Drawings

Somatic and spiritual aspects of children's drawings have not been as extensively researched as other aspects of children's art expressions. While most of the literature on children's drawings has focused on their creative work as representative of developmental and emotional influences, it is hard to ignore that children's drawings may contain other elements that cannot always be neatly classified within these categories. Arguably, somatic and spiritual aspects are two areas that overlap with other topics of this book. However, because they also present some unique dimensions of children's art expressions and are particularly meaningful in understanding images made by children who are experiencing life-threatening illnesses, coping with grief, or dying, somatic and spiritual aspects are important in their own right.

The term "somatic" is defined as of or relating to the physical body, distinct from the mind or the environment. Somatic aspects of children and their drawings may include characteristics that express or depict physical impairments or disabilities and acute or chronic physical illnesses. In the case of the latter, art expressions may reflect children's experiences with life-threatening illnesses or conditions such as cancer, heart, or kidney problems, surgery or invasive medical treatments, or serious traumatic injuries from accidents or abuse.

Spiritual aspects of children's drawings refer to content or characteristics that reflect children's experiences of God or intangible entities such as angels, religious figures, or ghosts and the supernatural, and experiences associated with church or religion. The term "transpersonal" is sometimes used in place of the word spiritual and is a term that has been used to describe phenomena beyond the personality and across cultures; it literally means "beyond the self." At other times the word "religious" is used to connote the spiritual aspects, but religion is actually only one expression of spirituality. For the purpose of this chapter, the term "spiritual" is used in order to encompass not only religious beliefs but also perceptions and experiences that relate to that which is beyond the self.

This chapter presents perspectives on how somatic and spiritual aspects are reflected in children's drawings. The first half of the chapter focuses on how children express physical illness, reactions to medical interventions and treatment, and beliefs about illness. The second half of the chapter examines how children include spiritual issues in their drawings, with an emphasis on children's experiences of life-threatening and terminal illnesses and grieving.

SOMATIC CONDITIONS EXPRESSED IN CHILDREN'S DRAWINGS

In Chapter 2, I described an 8-year-old girl who consistently drew black shapes in the center of each of her figures in her drawings. During the course of therapy, she eventually verbalized that the black markings were related to the physical pain she was experiencing in her stomach, a symptom she did not talk about in order not to be a burden to her family. Like many children from abusive homes who are primarily concerned about other members of their family rather than themselves, the girl felt that she could not talk about the physical pain she was experiencing. Her repetitious use of black in her drawings became a way to talk about her feelings and concerns, particularly the physical symptoms she was reluctant to express. Although not every rendition of black in the center of a figure will mean physical pain or illness, it is an unusual characteristic and one that may relate to a somatic condition. My experience in working with this girl was a turning point in my work as an art therapist because previous to this time I never considered the possibility that art expressions might also reveal or reflect somatic or physical conditions.

Although there are relatively few authors who have explored the topic of somatic conditions expressed in children's drawings, there is some precedent for understanding children's images from this perspective. Lowenfeld (1947) (see Chapter 4), was one of the first to note the appearance of children's physical impairments in drawings of human figures. He observed that repeated exaggeration or distortions of the same body part or area of the figure by children with physical problems often pointed to a defect or "abnormality" within the body. For example, a child who experienced paralysis on one side of the body might reflect it through a shorter leg or arm on one side of a self-portrait. Or a child with a broken arm may give that arm some sort of emphasis in a drawing, either by enlarging it or accentuating it with color. Although children may emphasize a particular feature in their figure drawings in response to a physical condition, it is also important to remember that children may exaggerate aspects of their drawings for other reasons. In looking at drawings, the therapist needs to be aware that any distortion may have either developmental or emotional origins, or may simply be the result of the creative or artistic license of the child.

Uhlin (1979), like Lowenfeld, noted that physically impaired children may portray aspects of their conditions in their art expressions. He believed that at least part of their portrayal involves their responses to their impairments as well as the impairment itself. In other words, children react in a variety of ways to physical impairments or conditions, and these reactions present themselves in their drawings. In his work with children with neurological impairments, Uhlin observed characteristics in children's drawings that he thought were indicative of their physical conditions, particularly in what he termed "body-image projections." Like Lowenfeld, he observed a number of drawings of children with neurological and other impairments who used either exaggeration or omission to express both conscious and unconscious feelings about the impaired parts of their bodies.

Martorana also observed that the type of drawing directive given to children with physical impairments may influence the outcome. For example, when asked to simply "draw a man," children with orthopedic problems overwhelmingly drew normal figures (in Uhlin, 1979). But when the same population was asked to draw a self-portrait, three-fourths of the children drew their impairments by exaggerating or distorting a body part, or reflected the impairment through omission. This finding underscores the impact of the type of drawing directive (in this case, draw a man vs. draw a picture of yourself) on the content of image, at least with regard to physical characteristics.

In cases of physical impairment, the therapist often knows in advance that a particular child has a physical condition or disability, and it is easier to make connections about it through the child's drawings. In situations where children are ill with cancer, renal failure, heart problems, or other serious conditions, less is known about how children express themselves through drawing. Drawings are thought to provide therapists with information on children's perceptions of pain or symptoms that are difficult to express through words; reactions to medical interventions; surgery, or drug treatment, and possibly trends in health, recovery, or physical deterioration (Malchiodi, 1993).

Susan Bach (1966, 1975, 1990) is one of few individuals who looked at seriously ill children's art expressions for what they may contain in terms of somatic information. Bach, a psychoanalyst, became interested in the spontaneous drawings of children and began investigating the use of painting as a way to understand emotional conflict. She realized the potential for understanding children from a multidimensional perspective, including physical aspects, noting that "not only the mental and psychological state was reflected but also the condition of the body" (Bach, 1990, p. 8) and that

> free paintings may reflect specific physical illnesses in typical colors, shapes, motifs, etc. They can show present acute states and point back to past traumatic events. Often ahead of recognized symptoms, they may indicate the future development of an illness, even asymptomatic processes, which, at the time, cannot be diagnosed. (1975, p. 87)

Although Bach's work remained focused on art expressions as diagnostic tools rather than for their therapeutic value, she did provide a major contribution in the area of understanding children's art expressions from a somatic perspective.

Later Furth (1988), who was intrigued with Bach's research, emphasized that somatic conditions may be covertly expressed through children's spontaneous drawings weeks or months before the condition is actually diagnosed. Like Bach, Furth notes that drawings may contain content that forecasts illness, recovery, and prognosis. Furth's work with what he calls "impromptu drawings" also underscores that many aspects of a child's experience may be present in an art expression and that it is important to not only pay attention to intrapersonal and interpersonal information but also to the possibility of somatic conditions appearing in drawings.

In my own work with medical populations, I have noticed that children do seem to express their physical conditions intuitively through their drawings. They also often record their reactions to medical procedures such as surgery, radiation, or drug treatment in their drawings. Many children undoubtedly express their fears, anxieties, or other feelings about being operated on, receiving chemotherapy or radiation treatments, or painful interventions. However, other children express experiences more directly related to the physical aspects of their conditions. For example, a 7-year-old child who had a kidney transplant drew herself with a kidney attached to the flank of her torso (Figure 7.1). Not all children who have had surgery will depict their experiences in this way after their transplant operation, and why some do include it is not known. In my experience, those children who include characteristics related to a surgery or procedure may be actively seeking to communicate their fears, questions, or confusion about what has physically happened to them. In the case of another child with a kidney transplant, she was very concerned about what people would think about the scar on her body and her attractiveness to others, since she was just becoming a teenager when she had the transplant operation. She also had questions and concerns about a transplanted kidney and wondered about the implications of having someone else's organ in her body. Her drawing, like that of the 7-year-old, presented visual clues that could enable the therapist to intervene, in order to address her worries, perceptions, and fears.

In the course of treatment, most children hospitalized for physical illnesses receive some sort of drug treatment as a part of their medical intervention; this treatment may also have impact on the content and style of their drawings. The drawings of children with renal (kid-

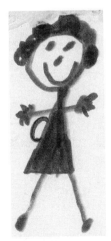

FIGURE 7.1. A 7-year-old girl's drawing of a person with a kidney attached to the torso.

ney) problems and related conditions have pointed to some interest-ing possibilities in the area of drug effects on this population. For ex-ample, the 13-year-old girl who had received a kidney transplant and was put on steroids after her surgery consistently drew pictures of her-self (Figure 7.2) and other people with enlarged heads. Steroid drugs can produce serious side effects, including swelling of the face and other parts of the body. It is important to remember that developmen-tally this characteristic (enlargement or exaggeration) may become less meaningful and more difficult to distinguish at stages in develop-ment when children naturally exaggerate features of their drawings to make a point or to accentuate something important in their drawing. However, in older children and adolescents (such as the girl described above) who generally draw more realistically and in proper propor-tion, this feature may be more significant and possibly related to the effect of the steroid medication.

COLOR AND SOMATIC CONDITIONS

Children's use of color in their drawings seems to be one characteristic that may have strong connections to somatic conditions. Perkins (1977) conducted a preliminary study comparing drawings of children ages 3 to 12 years who had life-threatening illnesses with those of

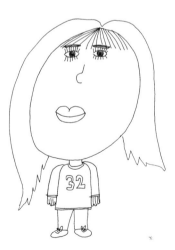

FIGURE 7.2. Self-portrait with an enlarged head by a 13-year-old girl who had a kidney transplant and was receiving steroid medication.

healthy children. The results of the study support the idea that children with serious illnesses do express both somatic and prognostic aspects in their art expressions, particularly through color. Perkins found that the drawings of the life-threatened children, the majority with cancer and a poor prognosis, contained color choices, symbols, and composition that were indicative of an awareness of impending death. In this particular study, the color black was used consistently by the children with serious illness. Perkins observed: "The black areas identified in the various pictures were generally consistent with negative affect in the children. Black was used to represent, among other things, a faceless nightmare creature, a cave, a vise, a spreading shadow, and a darkened house" (1976, p. 9).

The color red was used by both the control group (healthy children) and the life-threatened children, but the ill children used it more extensively, and their association to it was most often related to blood. Several others have mentioned red as a possible indicator of somatic conditions or as prevalent in the art expressions of children who are physically ill. For example, Bach noted red may be related to burning sensations, pain, or tumors and observed unusual uses of the color red by children with leukemia or other blood diseases. Levinson (1986), in her work with children who have been severely burned, observed that red and black were used to represent pain and trauma. In her clinical experience with children hospitalized for burns, if given the opportunity to paint a doll, they will invariably paint it with red or black on the areas of the body in which they have been burned.

In my experience in working with children with leukemia, I have found that the color red seems to play a prominent role in their drawings. For example, a 6-year-old girl recently hospitalized for treatment of her leukemia repetitiously drew a red sun freckled with red dots and an apple tree losing a great many red fruits (Figure 7.3). A 7-year-old boy drew a face he referred to as "the world" and covered it with red dots he called "bumps" (Figure 7.4). In his case, the red dots on the world may have had a prognostic element; two days later his face and arms were covered with small red hemorrhages, a characteristic of leukemia. Many leukemic children's drawings seem to include an unusual use of red markings, dots or jabs and, as Perkins (1977) also noted, frequent spontaneous depiction of fruit trees such as apple trees, often losing their fruits.

Bach (1990) felt that colors in children's art expressions had certain connotations, but she also emphasized the importance of "inten-

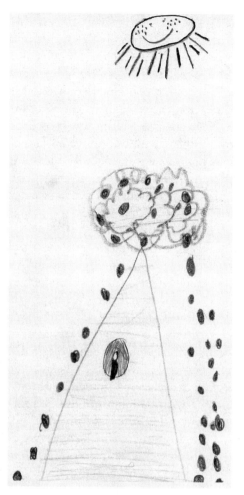

FIGURE 7.3. Drawing of a red sun with red dots and an apple tree losing its fruit by a 7-year-old girl with leukemia.

sity" of colors used. The term intensity refers to the vividness of color, its relative brightness or strength. For example, pink is a less intense color than bright red. With regard to children's drawings, although the color green may have universal connotations of growth and healing, whether the child used dark green or light green in his or her artwork may be more important when considering overall health or prognosis. A predominant use of dark green by a child in an art expression, according to Bach's research (Bach, 1990), would be more likely to be indicative of health or recovery, whereas light green may

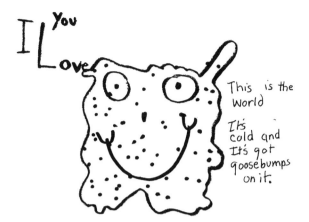

FIGURE 7.4. "The world" covered with red "bumps" by a 7-year-old boy with leukemia.

indicate that the child was physically weakened or, in some cases, coming back to health after medical treatment. In other words, any color may have various implications, depending on how it is used by the child in a drawing or painting.

CHILDREN'S BELIEFS ABOUT ILLNESS AND THEIR DRAWINGS

It may come as no surprise that children's personal concepts of what they believe illness to be are reflected in their art expressions. Banks (1990) conducted a study of how children perceive health and sickness, how colds happen, what germs are, and how medicine works with children from 3 to 15 years of age. A drawing task was used to evaluate children's understanding of "germs," the invisible entities that cause one to become sick. Three age groupings were created (3 to 5 years, 7 to 8 years, and 9 to 12 years) for the purpose of the study. Not surprisingly, developmental influences were apparent in each age level. The children in the youngest age group drew forms that contained scribbles or rudimentary figures, images that would be expected from very young children. Many of the older children in this group (5-year-olds) drew forms that they categorized as "monsters," human or animal-like faces or shapes that had nonhuman characteristics such as horns, spikes, or large, pointed teeth. Monsters were also popular with children ages 7 to 8 years, but more frequently, they drew images that looked like cells of some sort, demonstrating their growing knowledge of biology and health concepts. In the oldest group, ages 9 to 12 years, the large majority of the drawings of germs were of cells of one type or another. The drawings, along with the children's verbal interviews, provide evidence that children's concepts of illness go from external (monsters) to internal (actual disease-causing cells in the body), and their images of these external and internal causes change with age and exposure to information on how one becomes sick.

This study underscores an important point of using drawing in therapy with children who are physically ill. Since children's impressions of their illnesses reflect their conceptions of how the illness was caused, they also may reflect children's feelings and perceptions about why they got sick. Many children feel guilty about their illnesses, thinking that they did something bad in order to get sick. This is particularly true of young children who naturally see illness as a "monster" or punishment, but older children may also perceive illness from a similar perspective. For example, a 9-year-old boy with terminal bone cancer struggled with the question of why he was stricken with what is a horribly painful disease, stating on several occasions that the devil was punishing him for "bad things he did." During this time, he drew a series of images depicting a devil torturing a cat on the operating table (Figure 7.5). In part, this drawing relates the intense physical pain the boy experienced as a result of bone cancer as well as some of the medical procedures used to treat his cancer, such as radiation and surgery. But another important theme is involved, one of punishment, not only punishment involving tortuous pain, but pain specifically inflicted by the devil.

Drawings can be useful, not only as a record of children's perceptions and feelings about illness or medical procedures, but also as a place for the therapist to help the child to rehearse the future and, in this way, alter beliefs about illness and treatment. For example, if a child needs to have surgery, the therapist may help the child express issues and feelings about the medical procedure through drawings. In the case of the boy who depicted his medical intervention as a form of torture, the therapist was able to start a conversation with him about his treatment and to help him find ways to adjust to the medical procedures he found painful and frightening. When children have concerns about the source, treatment, or outcome of their pain (particularly reassurance that they do not have a life-threatening condition),

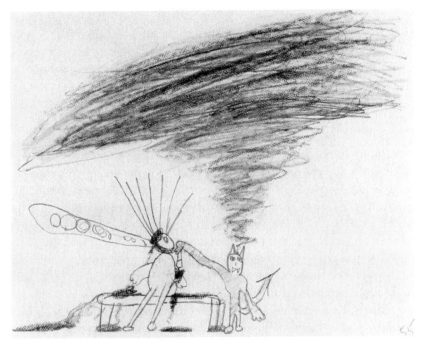

FIGURE 7.5. Drawing of the "Devil torturing a cat on the operating table" by a 9-year-old boy with bone cancer.

drawings that invite children to express their pain or symptoms can be helpful in understanding any questions, concerns, or fears that children may have.

The example of the little girl with the hidden duodenal ulcer described earlier underscores another significant point for therapists to consider in work with all children, whether they are ill or healthy. It can be important to ask children who have been traumatized, but have no obvious physical problems, where they think a certain feeling or emotion is located in their body (Malchiodi, 1982, 1990, 1997). For children who are worried about moving to a new home or seeing parents separate or divorce, children who have been abused or traumatized, or children who have experienced a death in their family, I have found that this is extremely helpful information in understanding where the child may develop psychosomatic problems later on or simply in knowing where the child feels emotional pain. To help children express this through drawing, I often give children a body image to color with markers, colored pencils, or crayons (Figure 7.6), showing me where the worry, fear, anger, sadness, or other emotion is in their bodies. Art therapists and other mental health professionals have developed tasks similar to this one in recent years (Gregory, 1990; Shoemaker, 1984; Steele et al., 1995). At the very least, children are able to begin to identify through this task where the trauma is felt in their bodies (head, tummy, heart) and how it is experienced (as an ache, a burning, a queasy feeling). This emphasis on the somatic aspects of their experiences of trauma or loss is an important component of using drawings as both intervention and evaluation. In many cases, the therapist may be alerted to any possible physical problems a child is having as a result of coping with trauma or loss. Certainly, in the case of the little girl with the ulcer, the stress she experienced as a result of her long-standing trauma severely affected her stomach. Her drawings of human figures, in particular, emphasized her physical pain through her repetitive use of color and, since she did not talk about her problem easily, were useful in revealing out that she had a serious medical condition.

With children who have an identified condition or illness, asking them to draw how they feel because of their illness or symptoms seems to be helpful in understanding how children personally experience physical problems. In some cases, it may even help the therapist or medical professional to develop a more accurate interpretation of the child's condition. In a study of children's headaches (Lewis et al., 1996), when asked to "draw a picture of how you feel when you have a headache," most children drew images that portrayed their symptoms, helping medical personnel to determine the classification of the headache (e.g., migraine, tension–vascular, or other type). In many

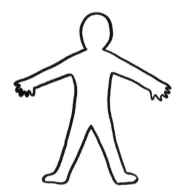

FIGURE 7.6. Example of body image exercise.

cases, children were able to communicate their specific symptoms more effectively through drawings than through words alone. For example, the quality of pain experienced was often differentiated through drawings: The children with migraines depicted images of pounding or hammering or throbbing, whereas those children with tension headaches included vices or belts around their heads in their human figure drawings. Although the sample of children studied was small, the trends in findings show promise in aiding understanding of children's somatic complaints through drawings as an adjunct to medical diagnosis.

SPECIAL CONSIDERATIONS IN WORKING WITH CHILDREN WHO HAVE PHYSICAL ILLNESSES OR IMPAIRMENTS

There are several overriding factors in using drawings with children who have physical impairments or conditions or are physically ill. First, it is important to realize that children who have physical conditions or illnesses may respond to drawing and art expression differently than children without physical impairments. Physical problems can and do affect children's abilities to participate in art making to varying degrees. For example, the children who are discussed in this chapter were often seriously ill, and their conditions certainly had an impact on their drawings in terms of detail, form, and content. In cases of serious illness, therapists must take into consideration that, for many sick or disabled children, drawing is almost impossible at times, due to pain, discomfort, or debilitation from either the illness, condition, or medical intervention. Children who might otherwise draw detailed images may resort to art expressions that are simple in form and content merely because they do not have the physical resources or stamina for art making that a healthy child would.

There are some overall considerations in choosing media and activities when working with children with physical illnesses or impairments and drawing. Attention should be given to the types of materials offered; for example, a child may find it more physically pleasurable to draw with a felt marker than a colored pencil, or vice versa, depending on what feels more comfortable. In order for some children who have physical disabilities to draw, the therapist may also have to make some adjustments to the materials, such as taping a drawing instrument to the child's hand or adapting the drawing surface to accommodate children who are bedridden or in a wheelchair.

The hospital environment in which most physically ill children are seen by therapists often requires some accommodation from both therapist and child. Working with children at their bedside, with medical equipment such IV bottles and monitors, poses some unique circumstances for art making. The bedtray may be the only surface available for the child to use as a support when drawing, and this too may be crowded with water containers and other items related to the hospital stay. Infection is also often a concern, particularly with children with compromised immune systems, open wounds, or severe burns. In these cases, it may be difficult to provide art activities that will not be hazardous to the patient, and the therapist may have to restrict materials to those that eliminate the risk of infection, both for the child and others. Offering the child drawing materials will not physically compromise the child patient in most cases, but in order to be safe, the therapist may need to provide a new set of crayons, markers, or pencils to each child to reduce the chance of exposure to and spread of contagious organisms.

Additionally, the constant onslaught of medical personnel checking children's vital signs or administering medication and family and friends visiting children in hospitals makes drawing and art making a public event, rather than a private therapeutic session. This poses a challenge to the therapist because these are inherent circumstances that make privacy impossible and disrupt the child's art process. It is sometimes a formidable task to find an appropriate time and space to allow children in hospitals to draw uninterrupted and to provide both therapist and child the privacy necessary to talk about the child's art expressions.

Children with physical illnesses or conditions may be depressed or nervous; some are physically exhausted by surgery, treatments, and being away from home for an extended period of time. Some are simply frightened by their surroundings and their illness, or concerned about their family's worries and anxieties about them. Fears, confusion, sadness, and other powerful emotions may cause some children to withdraw, and communication of any kind can be difficult. However, it is surprising that many children, in spite of their conditions, can become deeply involved in creative work, particularly with the support of the therapist. Drawing may be one of very few activities available to these children and can be a welcome relief and escape from the constant barrage of medical tests and interventions. Bach (1990) noted that art expression plays a compelling role in the expression of both spiritual and somatic aspects:

> The nearer some children, and also adults, come to a critical moment in their lives, the greater the urge to paint (should physical strength allow it). It seems that under the pressure of a life and death situation, hitherto untapped sources are activated and expressed. (p. 9)

This observation perhaps underscores the important role that art expression plays in work with seriously ill children, particularly those children who are life-threatened by their illnesses.

Finally, it is important to realize that it may be difficult or impossible to clearly identify characteristics of drawings as either having somatic or emotional origins. The little girl who used the color black to portray her painful ulcer certainly could be expressing the deep emotional pain she experienced as a result of living in a violent family. The child who included the marking on the body drawing may have also been expressing her fears and anxiety about her altered body image as a result of surgery and transplantation. Therapists who work with children with physical illness or impairments generally know about their patients' medical condition. With this information in mind, at times it is very difficult to be objective when looking at children's drawings and not to read more than there really is in the drawing in terms of physical illness or symptoms.

SPIRITUAL ASPECTS
OF CHILDREN'S DRAWINGS

Spiritual aspects of children's drawings have received relatively little attention when compared to other areas of children's art, for several possible reasons. It is well-known that Freud, whose work influenced the practice of psychiatry and psychology for most of this century, was not favorable to the subject of spirituality in his writings. Jung, although far more sympathetic to the concept of spirituality than Freud, felt that spiritual experiences were the province of the second half of life, not childhood. Although the idea that spiritual aspects are important to therapy has gained increasing acceptance over recent years, many therapists still shy away from including or recognizing these issues in their work with children.

Robert Coles's (1990) extensive work with children and his explorations of children's "spiritual lives" through both verbal interviews and drawings has renewed interest and curiosity in understanding children's perceptions and expressions of spiritual experiences. Although some question exists as to whether children actually have spiritual experiences in the same sense that adults do, his work provides evidence that children do think about and experience spiritual matters, particularly in the form of religious beliefs and ideas about God, heaven, the devil, and angels, and the spiritual world of ghosts and the supernatural. Coles' interest in this area was inspired by his early work with children on iron lungs in Boston, children who, despite overwhelming circumstances, could find meaning in their lives and had surprisingly strong spiritual beliefs and convictions. This experience convinced Coles that children's personal religious and spiritual lives were a significant part of his clinical understanding and are important to clinical work with children in general. Over the course of his research, Coles interviewed more than 500 children about their spiritual lives through conversation and drawings, concluding that children, not unlike adults, asked and considered many of the same questions that adults ask about spiritual issues.

Kübler-Ross (1983) notes that children as young as age 3 or 4 can talk about their dying, are aware of impending death, and frequently use symbolic means such as drawing to convey their experiences. Kübler-Ross's therapeutic work with dying children has contributed to the knowledge of children's spirituality, based on years of work with dying people. Spiritual aspects of children's art expressions can encompass many things including religious symbols, images of spirits, ghosts, or representations of a deceased person. It is important for therapists to support and make it safe for children to convey their ideas about God and other spiritual entities, religion, and death, if only to allow them to explore through art expressions questions that they may have about life.

The following section presents some perspectives on how spiritual aspects may appear in children's art expressions. Whether or not this perspective will be useful to readers is dependent on personal beliefs and more importantly, an acceptance of the importance of spiritual aspects of children's experiences. Many therapists do not believe that children are capable of spirituality in any form, favoring the idea that the period of formal operations must be reached and abstract thinking achieved before spirituality is possible. Up until that time it is thought that children's thinking about death is concrete and is largely influenced by the religious beliefs of their families. Others do not believe that issues of spirituality are appropriate to therapeutic work with children and therefore would probably not find it useful to look at drawings for spiritual issues. Some therapists may even be uncomfortable with the topic of spirituality because they have not sorted through their own beliefs and do not feel that they can or should relate to children in this way.

It is my personal bias to include spirituality, spiritual beliefs, and religion as important to my understanding of and work with children, particularly in terms of the integral perspective I described earlier in this book. While drawings that include religious or spiritual themes could be understood from an emotional and developmental standpoint, it can be important to look at them through a slightly different lens. The drawings of children who are facing life-threatening illness and children who have lost a loved one described in the remainder of this chapter are particularly important to consider in terms of spiritual issues. Although all children may express ideas or perceptions that relate to spirituality or religious beliefs, these circumstances seem particularly relevant to spiritual aspects of drawings, possibly because the crisis of death naturally brings children face to face with questions about God, religion, and what happens when life ends.

CHILDREN'S EXPRESSIONS OF TERMINAL ILLNESS, DEATH, AND DYING

Serious or terminal illnesses bring an experience of profound trauma to children, including confrontation with the process of dying. Children may not be able to express their feelings and needs through words alone, but they may be able to relate unexpressed fears, questions, or anxieties through drawings. Seriously ill children need help in sorting out what is happening to them not only on a physical level (e.g., surgery, body changes, or effects of drugs), but also what is occurring on deeper, more existential levels. They often have questions about spiritual matters such as God, heaven, or angels, and may explore ideas through drawings about what will happen to them when they die. Children who have lost a parent, sibling, or significant person in their lives may also use art to explore and express themselves in similar ways.

There has been some question as to the depth of understanding that children have about death and dying. As previously mentioned, some believe that fully understanding the concept of death is not possible in early childhood and may not be accessible until the time of formal operations (Piaget, 1959) in early adolescence. Before that time, children are believed to go through specific stages in their understanding of death and dying. For example, 3- to 5-year-olds who are at the pre-operational period do not understand that death is final, seeing it as reversible and as a form of separation. Older children (5 through 9 years) see death as the result of cause and effect: They may see it as a consequence of doing something bad or evil. By age 9 or 10, children may be able to comprehend death as being irreversible and an inevitable outcome of life and to understand that it is the result of illness or other circumstances that affect body function (Wass, 1984).

Others are convinced that even very young children perceive and understand a great deal about death and dying and that children have similar spiritual questions about death as adults do. Kübler-Ross (1983) observed that children have an "inner knowledge of death," particularly through symbolic representations such as dreams and art expressions. She notes:

> If people doubt that their children are aware of a terminal illness, they should look at the poems or drawings these children create, often during their illness but sometimes months before a diagnosis is made. . . . It needs to be understood that this is often a pre-conscious awareness and not a conscious, intellectual knowledge. It comes from the "inner, spiritual, intuitive quadrant" and gradually prepares the child to face the forthcoming transition, even if the grown-ups deny or avoid this reality. (p. 134)

Kübler-Ross's observation underscores the idea that therapeutic work with life-threatened or terminally ill children and bereaved children demands that children's expressive work be understood from a different viewpoint. The experience of profound grief due to loss of a loved one such as a parent or sibling or the process of facing one's own death are two situations that require the therapist to understand children and their art expressions beyond emotional and developmental aspects. In particular, children's inner confrontation with unfinished business, struggles and questions about leaving life, and acceptance of the process of dying can be conveyed through creative activities such as drawing.

In my first year of work as an art therapist, I had an experience with a preadolescent girl that enriched my thinking about what children express through art, particularly with regard to spiritual issues. Sarah, a gifted 13-year-old student in an alternative school, went into a deep depression over the sudden death of her grandfather. She and her grandfather had been very close; the girl was actually closer to the grandparent than to her parents, who were busy professionals. Her grandfather served the role of both mother and father, as well as grandparent, and when he died suddenly, his death created a great loss in the girl's life.

After several months of grieving, Sarah came into an art therapy session with me with a small painting she had done on notebook paper earlier that day (Figure 7.7). She depicted what she said was a powerful dream she had had the night before the session. In the dream, her grandfather appeared in a large chair surrounded by all of his relatives, children, and grandchildren, with Sarah sitting to his right. In the dream, her grandfather gave everyone a blessing and told Sarah that he would be leaving her and that he realized that she would be all right now. Sarah then saw a reindeer come down from the sky and lead her

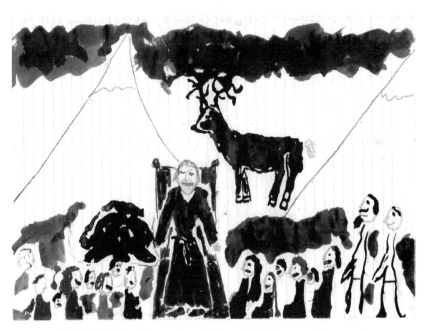

FIGURE 7.7. "Dream of my dead grandfather" by a preadolescent girl.

grandfather away. She was surprised by what she described as a "wonderful feeling of peace" this dream gave her but was equally perplexed at the appearance of the reindeer that came to take her grandfather away. Despite the sense of confusion, she felt comforted by the image of the reindeer and this experience and was able to put aside much of her grief over the loss of her beloved grandparent.

This dream and its contents present some of the more intangible aspects of imagery and depict an experience that goes beyond the self. While from an emotional perspective the image of the reindeer in Sarah's dream could be seen as a way to self-soothe and resolve the crisis of the grandfather's death, its qualities also speak of issues related to Sarah's perceptions of spiritual matters and experiences. Her dream image convey her impressions of how she perceived death and the idea of an afterlife after death. Her simple drawing poignantly shows her strong relationship with her grandfather and her feelings of resolution and is rich in metaphor that words cannot adequately describe.

Although very little has been written on the drawings of children who have lost a close relative or loved one, specific forms, colors, and content in the art expressions of life-threatened or dying children may provide some basis for recognizing and understanding spiritual aspects. Bach (1966, 1975, 1990), who believed that both body and soul were expressed through art, noted a specific configuration of elements that may appear in the drawings of children close to death. She observed that children begin to direct attention in their expressive work to the upper-left-hand section of the paper, perhaps including a road or pathway leading to that area. According to Bach, this area of the paper represents the movement of the sun to the west at the end of the day and for dying children, may represent leaving life. Bach felt that the upper-left-hand portion or quadrant of a drawing or painting held special significance in relation to spiritual issues and children's experiences of death and dying. Perkins (1977) in her work with terminally or life-threatened children also noted the appearance of a sun in the upper-left-hand corner of their drawings more than in those of healthy children.

After first reading about Bach's theory, I was skeptical that a specific section of children's drawings could be related to their experiences of dying. However, in work with cancer and AIDS patients, I have observed that both children and adults who are in the last few weeks or months of their lives, often include movement to this left-hand section or a light (sun or moon) in the upper-left-hand portion of their drawings. Sarah, the girl who was grieving her grandfather, explained that her reindeer was leading her grandfather to the upper-left-section of the drawing. While this may have been coincidence, one could also suppose that this too could be connected to Bach's theory that the upper-left area of the paper is a place of "going out of life."

Other elements have been noted in dying children's drawings that could be related to spiritual or transpersonal aspects of their experiences. For example, both Bach (1966) and Perkins (1977) observed the inclusion of a window in the eaves of house drawings by dying children. Bach refers to this as a "soul window," a small, often round window placed on roof or eaves of the house drawing. In Swiss folklore, the soul window is thought to be the place through which the recently deceased person leaves a house. Although there is no similar story in the United States, Perkins (1977) reports life-threatened children also included such windows in their house drawings.

Several other images have been mentioned in relation to dying children's drawings. Perkins (1977) noted the appearance of snakes in drawings, observing that they may connote transformation as well as the threat of serious danger to the self. Figure 7.8, a drawing by a girl with terminal leukemia, depicts a snake who she says "is carrying a mountain in the rain." In this case, the snake has a heavy, almost impossible burden that must be carried through inclement weather. At the time the child made the drawing, she was going through medical treatment that she realized would probably not help her. She had begun a final transformation through acceptance of her terminal condition, knowing that the doctors could not cure her and a few weeks later, died. In this picture, the snake is wearing glasses, a detail that she included in many of her drawings, including self-images, even though she did not wear glasses. The girl's eyes had become sensitive to light as a result of her leukemia, making it difficult for her to see distant objects.

As with the content of any drawing, it is important to ask children to describe or tell a story about their images (see Chapter 3). Although images in the drawings of dying children may hold special significance related to their experiences, many of these are common in healthy children's art expressions and as with most images, it is difficult to categorize them universally into one area of meaning. What is particularly important, however, is to take a nonjudgmental stance, allowing children to feel accepted for creating what may be sensitive and often heart-wrenching images and to explore questions they may have about death and dying through their drawings. As a result of his

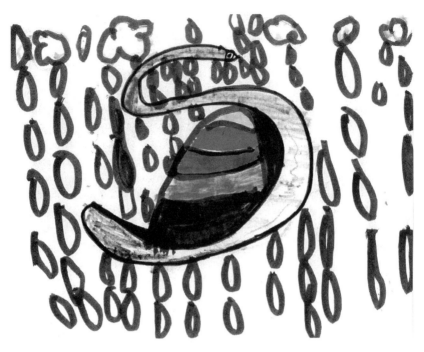

FIGURE 7.8. "Snake carrying a mountain in the rain" by a 7-year-old girl with leukemia.

work with seriously ill children, Allan (1988) observes, "a basic caring and a willingness to be open to the child's view will enable many to be effective in aiding a child on a journey through life" (p. 115) and, in the case of a dying child, through death.

Spiritual issues that dying children may express through drawing may be difficult for therapists, but they must be recognized and supported. Bach (1990) has some important advice for therapists who work with children who are seriously or terminally ill, noting:

> After all our endeavors to see the child's or parent's side, I feel very strongly that we need to look at those who surround the patient, including ourselves, and to assess our stamina and ability to stand the strain of what might be seen and realised in such a picture.
>
> This calls for considerable awareness of the difficulty of the work we are doing in studying seriously ill children's painting; it is important to learn how to feel with the child without becoming identified with his or her particular situation. (1990, p. 147)

Bach underscores the powerful impact that children's drawings, particularly those from children who are sick or dying, can have on helping professionals. Children's drawings of their struggles with illness may reflect profound pain and suffering, declining health, and the process of dying, issues that are very difficult to confront, but are important ones to address in therapeutic work with children with serious physical illness.

CONCRETE EXPRESSIONS OF SPIRITUALITY AND RELIGION

Aside from composition and content in children's drawings, many children will express spiritual beliefs concretely, including religious practices and concepts, through their drawings. For example, children may depict religious activities such as prayer, finding comfort in practices that they have been taught as part their family's religion. Other children may depict a dead relative as an angel (Figure 7.9) while very young children may fear that the ghost of a deceased person will come back or appear in their bedrooms (Figure 7.10). In the case of the latter, the child, a 4-year-old boy, worried that he had wished that his younger brother would die. Subsequently, when his brother did die, it caused him to become guilty and fearful. Children sometimes believe that wishing for something bad to happen to a person has magically caused the death, and this can result in profound guilt. When children express such beliefs through drawing, they often come in the form of ghosts or demons and are particularly important to recognize and acknowledge. As discussed in the section on somatic aspects expressed in drawings, some children see their illness as a punishment, feeling disciplined by God or the devil (see Figure 7.5) for doing something bad in the past.

Although dying children have been the focus of much of this section, it is important to realize that children in severe crisis because of abuse, trauma, or loss may express their experiences in ways that reflect spiritual or existential questions. For example, a girl whose father severely abused her and her younger sister drew an image of a heart with a knife through it, asking the question "Why did God do this to me?"

Other children may wonder through their drawings where dead people go or explore what form they take after death. A young Mor-

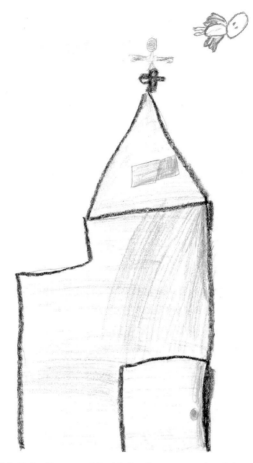

FIGURE 7.9. Drawing of dead father flying over a church by a 7-year-old boy.

mon child depicted her dead father as the same as other family members, based on the religious teachings of her faith, which convinced
her that someday she would again see her father as she remembered
him (Figure 7.11). One boy whose brother had died in an accident
used the color black to indicate his dead sibling, wondering out loud
to the therapist if his brother was now an angel with wings in heaven.
Grieving children do not always ask for help with their grief through
words, and art expressions may be one of few ways through which they
express their fears, anxieties, and confusion.

Questions about death that children may visually explore
through their drawings include: Where do I or other people go when

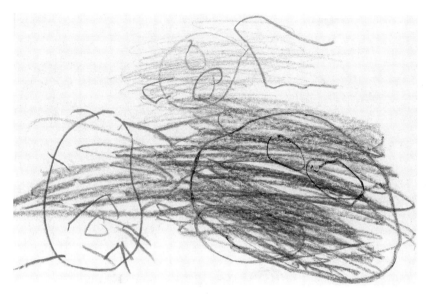

FIGURE 7.10. Drawing of his younger brother as a ghost by a 4-year-old boy; the ghost is the figure in the upper half of the drawing.

they die? Can my dead mother see me from heaven? Do dead people ever come back? It is obvious that the therapist should not have any particular religious stance in responding to these questions, but should be unbiased in allowing children to explore these concerns. Children will generally develop answers that match their cultural and family belief system.

Coles (1990) provides an important rationale for respecting and recognizing the spiritual aspects of children's drawings, observing that "children try to understand not only what is happening to them, but why; in doing that, they call upon the religious life they have experienced, the spiritual values they have received, as well as other sources of potential explanation" (p. 100). Resiliency, the ability of children to rebound and recover from stressful events, is strongly linked to children's sense of spirituality, among other characteristics (Center for Children with Chronic Illness and Disability, 1996). While it may not be necessary to have a strong sense of religious or spiritual beliefs, it is still a powerful personal characteristic that therapists may become aware of through children's art expressions. When working with children who are struggling with illness or bereavement, recognizing and supporting these beliefs if they appear in drawings could, at the very

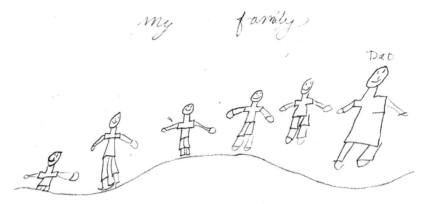

FIGURE 7.11. An 8-year-old girl's drawing of her dead father as he would appear someday in "heaven."

least, be important factors associated with helping children to cope with life-threatening physical conditions or to understand and assimilate a loved one's death.

CONCLUSION

In work with children who are seriously ill or confronted with death, it is important to remember that both somatic and spiritual elements are often present in their drawings. Noting the contributions of Bach and her work with dying children, Furth (1981) supports the notion that physical and spiritual aspects are inevitably connected, observing that that both body and spirit "act conjointly to serve the life and health of the individual . . . we should find this link expressed in the undirected, impromptu drawings of children" (p. 67), particularly the drawings of children who are seriously ill or dying. In this sense, drawings are a way to assist therapists more fully to understand life-threatened children, to allow them to communicate their experiences of serious illness and confrontation with death, and to be able to help these children "restore harmony between body and soul" (Furth, 1981, p. 69).

CHAPTER EIGHT

Ethical Considerations and Children's Drawings

The idea that the subjects of ethics and children's drawings are connected may surprise some therapists who use art activities as part of their work with children. With the exception of art therapists, most therapists who ask children to draw as a part of therapy or evaluation have not been trained or exposed to the specific ethical issues involved in handling art expressions created by child clients.

Children's drawings and other creative works are often visually engaging, intriguing, and charming, making it easy to forget that their images may also contain material that must be protected and that rights of choice, ownership, and privacy must be respected. In my own work as a therapist, there are many art expressions whose content is visually compelling, images that seem to cry out to be shared with others, especially to other professionals and caregivers who could benefit from understanding the children who created them. Deeply emotional content, untold family problems, and heart-wrenching stories are poignantly depicted through drawing by some children, particularly those children who have experienced trauma, abuse, loss, or crisis in their lives. Many of the drawings in this text have forceful messages or content. However, each image required serious ethical consideration before it was chosen to illustrate a point or idea. This includes confidentiality and display of art expressions; issues of ownership or disposition of the image; storage and treatment of art expressions; and safety for both the child and the child's creative work.

CONFIDENTIALITY AND DISPLAY
OF CHILDREN'S DRAWINGS

First and foremost, issues of confidentiality must be taken into account when working with children's drawings made during the course of therapy. Confidentiality is an ethical issue that is the basis of all therapeutic relationships and is defined as the responsibility to protect clients from unauthorized disclosure of information within the therapeutic relationship (Corey, Corey, & Callanan, 1993). While therapists, psychologists, and counselors may safeguard what children say in therapy or counseling, drawings are not always recognized as confidential communications. In actuality, many hospitals, agencies, and facilities do not see art expressions as private material. Client verbal records, audiotapes, and videotapes are routinely kept in locked files, but in many cases, art expressions are not regarded in a similar fashion because they are, for the most, part nonverbal. Also, since the language of art is extremely personal, many therapists believe that messages and content in art expressions are disguised and are not easily interpreted or understood by others who may see the work.

In writing this book, I had to make a great many difficult decisions about whether or not to include specific children's drawings. Some of the determinations to publish certain drawings were fairly easy; the children who created them were healthy, happy, and well-adjusted and were excited to know that their drawings would be published. Their artwork revealed nothing more than normal developmental characteristics and positive experiences. Others, however, were very difficult to choose, with a great many variables influencing decisions. In some cases, drawings that depicted unique situations, events, or experiences that could compromise the identity of the child had to be withheld. Some drawings, although useful as illustrations, were impossible to include because permission had not been received from a parent or guardian and the child to share the child's art. Other drawings, although consent was obtained, were just too personal to present; the disclosure of the experience through drawing in therapy with me was an experience that needed to be respected, despite what readers could learn from the images.

The use of drawings within any therapeutic framework does present some unique situations with regard to confidentiality that many therapists may not have considered. For example, although therapists can alter biographical information and names to disguise client identities, the uniqueness of art expressions cannot easily be changed to protect a client's privacy (Wilson, 1987). Some drawing styles can be as unique as one's handwriting. The situation becomes complicated if a child's art is exhibited with permission in a public place where relatives or friends may recognize the work, even when the artist's name is removed. Some images, for example, may reveal very specific information about the child, information that could compromise the child's or the family's well-being. The common request to draw a picture of one's family usually results in a picture that provides recognizable details; similarly, a request to draw a picture of a traumatic event might also provide details and characteristics that others may recognize.

Some of the confusion and unfamiliarity about the protection of drawings as confidential expressions comes from the nature of artistic expression itself: Art is often created with eventual display in mind. Children themselves frequently expect that the artwork they create will be displayed—their drawings made during a classroom art class are usually exhibited on bulletin boards or classroom hallways for others to see and admire. Art is usually made to be shared and viewed by others, a natural outcome of making visual images. For many children, seeing their work displayed where others can enjoy it is a very positive experience.

Some art expressions are created by children in settings outside therapy, such as a classroom, an art class, or even at home, and are not subject to the same concerns about confidentiality as those made in an individual therapeutic session. However, art made as part of therapeutic treatment intensifies the importance of issues of confidentiality and privacy regarding display. These expressions may contain material that, if publicly disclosed, may not be in the child's best interests and perhaps be dangerous to the self or others (Knowles, 1996; Malchiodi & Riley, 1996).

Children who have been or are suspected of being abused often require special treatment and ethical consideration of their drawings, and helping professionals must be particularly sensitive to their need for confidentiality. Art made in therapy may contain content that is not appropriate for the public to see, especially when a child expresses specific details about violent, abusive, or traumatic events that have occurred. In some cases, it is not advisable for art expressions to go home with the child who made them. For example, what if the art blatantly reveals that abuse by a parent has taken place, but protective services has not yet intervened on behalf of the child? Letting the child take home an art expression with material that would endanger the child's safety and well-being is obviously not appropriate. For this reason alone, careful thought must be given to the disposition of art expressions made by children whose lives may be compromised through further abuse or maltreatment.

This is one of many examples of why it is imperative to consider how art expressions made in therapy will be handled and how the rights of children will be protected with regard to the content and confidentiality of their art. This example also reinforces the necessity to establish a procedure to inform children at the outset of therapy (see preceding section on confidentiality for more information) that there may be some circumstances when it is important for the therapist to retain their art, especially in cases where the child may be subjected to abuse or violence because of the content. Explaining to the child why certain art expressions will be retained also indicates that the therapist respects the child and his or her art product.

Because children's art expressions, especially those made by children in distress, are so visually compelling, hospitals and clinics often want to exhibit them to draw attention to children's issues such as abuse or trauma. Although these exhibitions of children's work may have the best intentions, this practice may not be in the best interests of children. I am sadly reminded of an annual exhibition of children's drawings and paintings that a large residential treatment program stages in my home state. The works of art exhibited were a result of a therapeutic art class that children attend as part of their psychiatric rehabilitation. Although the staff of the program felt that it was appropriate to publicly exhibit the children's work, the art expressions were also displayed to call attention to the hospital's programs and staff, and to solicit funding for the facility. Unfortunately, much of the art exhibited was very revealing and highly emotional in content. To add to the problematic aspects of the situation, several of the children who created the art were interviewed on the local TV news, thus compromising their confidentiality and privacy.

Children's art is sometimes used by facilities and the media in this way because it is often visually touching and colorful, and naturally draws attention and public interest. However, therapists who decide to make children's more sensational art expressions public through exhibition also have to consider if this practice is in the children's best interest or promotes interests other than those of the children. Therapists and the agencies must respect the child's overall safety and well-being, and be concerned primarily with the protection of the child clients they seek to help. Unfortunately, some facilities display children's art expressions as part of publicity campaigns to draw attention to their programs and hopefully generate donations for their services and programs. Although this type of display may serve to educate others about the art activities with children, it may is not always in the children's best interests. It seems somewhat ironic that children who may have emotional problems, are in crisis, or are recovering from abuse or trauma are also inadvertently abused through misuse of their art expressions by the same adults who want to intervene in their behalf.

It is also important to remember that when a child knows that artwork will be displayed in some public way, he or she may change the style, content, and tone of the drawing. If a child knows that his or her art will be displayed, the child may become more concerned with how the drawing looks and less free in expressing him- or herself. The question also becomes a therapeutic one: If children know that the work will be displayed, will they censor what they draw? In some cases, probably so, especially because children in therapy often seek the approval of others they perceive to be in authority.

In some circumstances, display of drawings can be as important as creating the drawings themselves, and there occasionally are situations when display overrides issues of confidentiality. For example, when I worked as an art therapist at a shelter for battered women and their children, I had the flu for several days and had to miss work. At the next art therapy session, in response to my absence, a group of children made pictures of monsters that would "grow tall and eat me up" if I should miss another meeting with them (Figure 8.1). Posting these drawings on the door to my office was an important aspect of the experience, since it was a public place where everyone else who worked at the shelter could see them, thus adding to my shame and serving as potent warning to me never to miss work (i.e., abandon these children) again. Although I usually would feel uncomfortable displaying the art expressions of children in a public place, it is easy to understand how some circumstances bypass the usual rules.

The display of art can be an important component of a children's therapeutic program, as demonstrated in the preceding example, and an effective way to support and strengthen a child's sense of identity and self-confidence. Most children who make drawings or art pieces are proud of their work and want to show it to others. Many times an

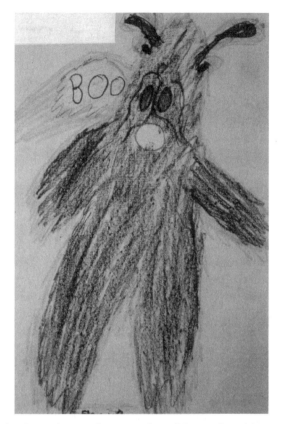

FIGURE 8.1. Crayon drawing of a monster that will "grow tall" and devour the therapist.

art activity is specifically designed to elevate self-esteem and encourage feelings of self-worth and pride, and displaying the finished work may support this goal. There are times when the therapists may need to consider displaying children's work not only from an ethical viewpoint, but also for its value as a therapeutic intervention. For example, it may be significant to children with tentative feelings of self-worth to share drawings they have created with others who can praise their efforts and abilities. In this way, art expression can serve as a source of pride for children when they may feel failure in other areas of their lives.

There are some ways that display of drawings can be accommodated without compromising children in treatment. If the facility has space that is not public and is secure, then selected work probably can be selectively and safely displayed. Sometimes the room where art therapy takes place is a good choice, especially if a large cork board or wall is available to use for hanging drawings or other flat work. In my own studio–office, I have a place where art can be displayed for at least the time the child comes to a session; for many children, it is important to see their work on my wall when they come in for their session. In some facilities, there are restricted areas that are for clients and staff only; if secure from anyone damaging or taking the art, this area is another possibility for display on a limited basis.

Many decisions to display will not be easy, and there are a few additional factors to consider in making a decision. Some children, although often initially excited by the idea of displaying their work to others, are not emotionally strong enough to handle what others say about their work. They may perceive even compliments as threatening, not being able to accept or understand positive remarks made about their art. Some parents may not understand the content of the art expressions and may react in a way that is counterproductive to supporting the child. In these cases, it is often beneficial for the therapist to educate the parents about how to respond to and talk with their children about their creative work. Some simple examples of what to say to children about their drawings, how to extend appropriate praise, or how to display drawings when they go home with children can be very helpful in extending the therapeutic gains made in therapy.

Lastly, no matter how art expressions are handled, therapists will want to develop appropriate forms for release of art expressions for educational purposes, for display, and for sharing with other professionals involved in the child's case (Malchiodi, 1996). Artwork should first and foremost be considered confidential statements from the child made while in therapy and treated accordingly.

OWNERSHIP

Ownership of drawings made by children in therapy or other settings may seem like a simple matter, and in most cases, ownership is not a problem. In the natural course of making art, the children who create the drawings or art expressions expect to keep the drawings they create, especially if they like to draw and feel positively about their creations. However, depending on what the purpose of the drawing is (assessment, evaluation, or treatment), the work may be retained by the therapist or psychologist as part of the permanent file of the child.

It is important for therapists to consider how they will handle ownership issues of art expressions created by the children they see. If drawings are retained as part of a child's file while that child is in treatment, the question of who owns the art must be addressed. Although it may seem that the child who created the art owns it, some think that in certain cases the therapist is responsible for it, since he or she has responsibility for the child. In other cases, the parents or guardians who are legally responsible for the child may feel the art work belongs to them, and, in some circumstances, the agency or facility where the drawing was completed as part of therapy may feel that the drawing belongs in their files. The question of ownership is not an easy one to answer, but is one that must be considered when using drawings as part of therapy.

Informed consent, the right of the client to be informed of the purpose, goals, and limitations of therapy, involves some unique ethical issues about children's ownership of the art they make in therapy. Issues of informed consent in therapy with children raise many general ethical questions: the extent of their competency to consent to or decline treatment, the role of parental consent and involvement, and disposition of records and other materials that result from therapy, including drawings. Since children are assumed by law to be incompetent, decisions involving therapeutic issues usually come from either parents or guardians. Confidentiality, for example, becomes a very difficult issue from the outset, since it is often impossible to separate the child's interests from those of consenting parents or guardians. Drawings and other art products that result from therapy could conceivably be seen as the property of the adults who brought the child into treatment; this is a question of both ownership and confidentiality not easily answered, but it is an issue that must be considered in certain circumstances.

When children are asked to leave their drawings with the therapist, other issues related to the therapist–child relationship may arise. Although children may agree to give the therapist their work for their files, internally they may feel differently, perceiving that something important was taken from them. They may not express these emotions openly to the adult in authority, fearing retribution, being afraid of being rejected, or simply wanting to please the therapist because they want to be praised in return. These dynamics are often particularly true of children who have been abused, neglected, or otherwise previously hurt by adults in their lives.

Luckily, most children do not seem to be attached to keeping drawings that are the result of assessment or projective drawing activities such as drawing a person or similar task. They generally understand that these tasks are more like tests rather than creative activities. However, other activities that involve using different materials with which to draw, paint, or sculpt are often perceived as pleasurable and may create more personal investment in the expression created. These art expressions may have more meaning, are more related to a sense of accomplishment, and bring with them a sense of self-esteem.

In many situations, I have worked with children who have told me that they wanted me to keep their drawings for them. Often these children have severe emotional trauma, have experienced profound crises, or have been subjected to physical or sexual abuse. Their drawings often contain painful feelings and memories; these images may be too distressing to take with them after creating them. In asking the therapist to keep these expressions, these children may experience a measure of safety from their own feelings and circumstances, seeing the therapist as a container for at least some of their pain, which they have expressed through art.

My personal view on ownership holds that if a child wants to keep an art expression, it is ethical and therapeutically sound to respect that child's prerogative. Photocopies can easily be made for the file or photos may be taken if needed. It is only in cases where the content of the art expression compromises the safety of the child or when the art expressions are utilized as evidence in court that the product must be retained.

SAFETY

The subject of safety touches on many of the issues already discussed in this chapter. Confidentiality, display of drawings, and ownership all involve aspects of safety to some extent. Providing safety, however, encompasses other dimensions in the area of ethics and children's art. Reflecting on her many years of work with children, Rubin (1984a) beautifully states the overall importance of safety in art therapy:

Safety means that many kinds of expressive activity are accepted: bizarre as well as realistic, regressive as well as progressive, those with negative as well as positive subject matter. Limits help to protect children from their own impulses, so that while it is safe to smear chalk or to draw destructive fantasies, it is not safe or permitted to smear people or to behave destructively toward property. In work with children, it is important to protect them from outer as well as inner psychological dangers, such as people and practices which would limit or stunt their creative growth. (p. 33)

The issue of safety also touches on what children are allowed to draw or create through art within a therapeutic or agency setting. Although children are generally encouraged to draw whatever they want, there are some circumstances when rules about what can be depicted may be a concern, and in some cases problems of censorship may arise (Haeseler, 1987). For example, in a psychiatric unit in which I worked, rules were established by the agency that restricted the content of drawings created by adolescent patients in art therapy. According to the guidelines created by the agency, patients were not allowed to draw violent images or subjects that contained satanic themes. These restrictions were particularly difficult for these adolescents who often drew pictures containing images from the current rock music groups, the content of which usually had violent or antireligion overtones.

Censorship of art expressions puts issues of safety into question from two perspectives. First, when there are rules about what can or cannot be expressed through drawings, free expression and what is "safe" or acceptable to express is brought into question. This practice becomes particularly problematic when it is imposed after the fact, and rules are created in response to the content of a particular child's drawings. For example, Haeseler (1987) notes that if initially told that one can draw whatever one wants, sudden imposition of rules about expression can result in feelings of anger and betrayal in children and adolescents.

On the other hand, violent imagery can be problematic especially if created within or as part of a group. The content of art can have a powerful effect on those who view it; children who are traumatized by physical or emotional trauma, have serious mental illness, or are emotionally frail for whatever reason may react strongly to seeing such images from other children. There are some circumstances when children may have to be protected from others' images during the process of art expression as therapy for their own safety and welfare.

Safety is important not only in terms of the child's experience of drawing and creative art activities but also in regard to how the child's drawings are handled. A therapist will quickly lose the trust of the child he or she is working with if drawings are lost, abused, or destroyed beyond repair. The child's work must be kept in a safe, secure place and with the idea that it will remain safe from harm or inappropriate inspection by others. Too often, therapists are not respectful of children's work, writing on it without permission of the child or allowing it to become tattered or damaged. This lack of concern for the "safety" of children's creative work sends a powerful message to them about a therapist's lack of respect for both their drawings and the children themselves.

Finally, it is important to reinforce issues of safety involved in the disposition of the drawings of children who have experienced abuse. As previously noted, these drawings must be handled carefully, with the utmost concern for children who have disclosed through drawings the details of physical or sexual abuse that occurred to them. In such situations, it is imperative that the drawing stays in a safe place and that it not go home with the child into circumstances which would compromise the child's safety should the disclosure be known.

STORAGE OF ART EXPRESSIONS

One of the most unwieldy aspects of children's drawings is their storage. Storage is needed for two purposes: (1) for children's confidential files that contain sample or significant drawings and expressions; (2) for art products-in-progress, paintings, or large drawings. At the very least, a locked storage area should be provided so expressions are given a secure place that is safe from theft or damage, or in order to protect privacy.

Storing or retaining drawings as part of children's files or for other reasons brings up both ethical and legal issues involving drawings as records of treatment. At least one ethical code, that of the American Art Therapy Association (AATA), has taken initial steps to explore the idea of drawings as treatment records. The AATA ethical document states that "art therapists shall maintain patient treatment records for a reasonable amount of time consistent with state regulations and sound clinical practice, but not less than 7 years from completion of treatment or termination of the therapeutic relationship. Records are stored or disposed of in ways that maintain confidentiality" (AATA, 1995).

It is difficult to say from reading this excerpt whether art expressions created during therapy are considered "treatment records" per se, or if they are, that they must be retained for the stipulated 7-year period. The majority of therapists would probably agree that the child who makes the drawing owns it. However, as already mentioned, it may also be true that in some instances artwork may constitute a medical or legal record and must be retained in a locked file or secure facility. Cases of abuse, trauma, or family violence are a few examples of circumstances when it may be necessary to retain and store children's drawings.

ETHICAL ISSUES AND THE USE OF PROJECTIVE DRAWING PROCEDURES WITH CHILDREN

Over the last decade, there has been considerable debate about the ethics of using projective procedures such as the Draw-A-Person Test (DAP), House–Tree–Person (HTP), and other drawing "tests" as ways to assess personality. The problems with these procedures, particularly in the area of reliability, are described in more detail in Chapter 1. Equally problematic are some of the more recent drawing tasks and protocols that are purported to be useful in assessment but have not been standardized and have not been fully researched (Malchiodi, 1994). However, since these protocols are often used to evaluate children, it is important to consider the ethics involved in using these tasks to assess and make inferences about the individual child.

First and foremost, the choice to use a specific projective or art-based assessment with a child should depend on the age of the child and the purpose for which the assessment will be used. Hopefully, therapists who use projective tasks with children have had personal experience (e.g., been a subject who has had the HTP, DAP, or other tests administered to them) with projective drawings. Therapists must also be aware of the most recent research on assessment and evaluation in order to use projective drawing protocols. Using drawings for evaluative purposes is a serious matter and therapists must be fully cognizant of what they are doing.

For the most part, projective drawing tests are used to make general observations about the personality of a child or to support generalizations from other sources such as rating scales, self-report measures, or therapist, teacher, and/or parent observations. Although scoring systems have been developed, in most cases, the results of these projectives are used to bolster results from other sources. Martin (1988) observes some reasons why this practice is inappropriate and possibly unethical. First, it implies that adding up responses to both projective drawing tests and other instruments is a reliable way to determine personality. Martin (1988) notes:

> If a child looks anxious in the testing situation, if his teacher rates him as anxious on a standardized rating scale, and the Draw-A-Person has provided one or two indices that could be interpreted as indicating the presence of anxiety, then the clinician feels comfortable about making the generalization that the child is anxious, and feels that the Draw-A-Person has been helpful in documenting the presence of the condition. (p. 3)

Martin also emphasizes the ambiguity and contradictory meanings associated with any one characteristic in the DAP test (e.g., meanings are associated with a drawing with a large head, omitting hands, or including buttons on a shirt). The possibility for multimeaning is intrinsic to art expression but creates an ethical problem for the therapist who uses this type of limited data to support a hypothesis about the personality of the child through characteristics of the drawing.

A final concern about the use of projective drawing tasks and the protocols used to analyze drawings is that information obtained from them can reinforce a bias that the clinician may have about the child, and the clinician will be pulled toward looking for characteristics that support his or her stance. For example, the clinician may stereotype the child as one who is defensive, finding evidence in the characteristics of the drawing that bolsters this supposition. Or, the clinician may use data obtained from the drawing task to ask others if the child seems defensive and, in turn, perhaps increases the chance of bias in their responses to the child.

I find using projective tasks and their respective protocols to be problematic for one reason: They utilize singular graphic characteristics to infer a particular personality trait or condition. Perhaps my training as an artist, art educator, and art therapist has sensitized me to one important aspect of art expression—its synergistic quality. All images are made up of many components—lines, shapes, form, composition, and color; what makes each unique is the endless ways that these qualities come together in a drawing or other art form. It is difficult at best to dissect a drawing into singular elements without losing sight of the overall content of the image and without becoming fixated on specific characteristics and sometimes missing others. While I do believe that it is possible to develop ways to rate aspects of drawings, many of the traditional projective drawing tests do not provide reliable ways of doing so and must be used carefully and with full knowledge of their limitations.

Given that many art therapists and other health professionals use art expressions not only to understand their clients, but also for assessment, evaluative, and sometimes diagnostic purposes, it is extremely important to have a complete understanding of the ethics involved in using art expressions in such a way. For some, the very question of using art expressions for assessment or diagnosis is an ethical one in and of itself. Also, given the minimal amount of research data available on the exact meaning of art expressions in general, it is still difficult to make a prediction from graphic data without additional information such as client statements or behaviors. Therefore, any use of art expression to assess or evaluate a child requires therapists be current in their knowledge of research data as well as sensitive to the use of art products to interpret the individual child.

LEGAL IMPLICATIONS FOR CHILDREN'S DRAWINGS MADE DURING THERAPY

At some point in working with a child, the art expressions created in therapy may become important sources of information for various reasons. One area involves legal actions, particularly those involving suspected physical or sexual abuse to children. Since drawings may provide evidence of serious problems in children, as with any material that results from therapeutic interaction, it is important to keep accurate records of drawings, and certainly crucial if one is using drawing as a central focus of therapy.

In my experience in training and supervising therapists in the use of art in therapy, many therapists prefer to document or record what the child says about the drawing directly on the image. Although this practice does offer convenience and perhaps accurate recording of data, it is ethically and perhaps legally problematic for several reasons. First, the issue of respect for the child's work is ethically important. Writing on the drawing may devalue the image; the child may feel disrespected for what she or he has created when words and notes are written directly on the drawing. The practice of writing on a drawing may also may interfere with how the image is viewed later on. If the drawing is later used in additional evaluation or as evidence in a court case, this may detract from its value.

Many therapists and attorneys have asked me if drawings can withstand scrutiny in a court of law, particularly children's drawings in cases of abuse or domestic violence, or violent crime. Since children who are traumatized by physical or sexual abuse or similar trauma often do not want to talk or cannot articulate with words the details of their experiences, it is natural to think that their drawings might be able to convey information important to understanding their situations and to their welfare and safety. If a child's life or welfare is endangered, art expressions, particularly those made as part of therapy, may become part of evidence should the legal system or child protective services be involved. However, to my knowledge, it is quite difficult to rely solely on children's drawings to reliably convey information on abuse or trauma, largely because the research on indications of abuse or trauma in drawings is still inconclusive.

Despite the lack of conclusive data on the content of children's drawings, their use in court is still an important area to consider. Drawings fall into a category known as "novel scientific evidence" (Cohen-Liebman, 1994). Although there is some research to support graphic characteristics of trauma, violence, and emotion in children's work, over all, the research is still not completely reliable. Due to the nature of art expressions themselves, it may never be completely possible to determine from the content of a child's drawings elements of the child's experiences. However, children's drawings still may be admitted as evidence in court by passing specific admissibility tests of the court in order to determine validity of the evidence.

It is more likely that the qualifications of the therapist who serves as an expert witness concerning the content of the drawings will determine their value as evidence. For example, in 1985, expert testimony from an art therapist was admitted after careful scrutiny of the therapist's qualifications to practice therapy and assessment involving art expression and her ability to give expert advice on the content of children's drawings (Levick, Safran, & Levine, 1990). The implication in this decision is that training and professional experiences with children's drawings are key to the use of art expressions as judiciary aids.

CONCLUSION

There is one final overriding caveat in using drawings to understand children: It is the responsibility of the therapist, counselor, psychologist, or teacher using drawings as aids to understanding children to continue to keep abreast of the wealth of information on children's drawings that continually becomes available. It is hoped that this book has given the reader a good start in understanding the multidimensional aspects of children's drawings and has provided a foundation for sensitivity to the content of children's art expressions in general. However, this is only a beginning, and in working with children's art expressions, it is the ethical responsibility of therapists to maintain their skills in this area in order to be of best service to the children they seek to help.

Rubin (1984a) eloquently articulated the cautions inherent in working with children and their drawings in therapeutic settings:

> Art is a powerful tool—one which like the surgeon's, must be used with care and skill if it is to penetrate safely beneath the surface. . . . The use of art with all kinds of children as a symbolic communicative medium is a clinically demanding task, which carries with it both a tremendous potential and an equally great responsibility. (p. 299)

Drawing undeniably offers children a potent and creative method of communicating themselves to helping professionals who work with them, whether in clinical settings, hospitals, shelters, or schools. How we, as helping professionals, respond to children's drawings and encourage and appreciate these creative expressions not only gives them value in assessment and treatment but also provides a framework for understanding, respect, and regard for the children who have been generous in their sharing of their creative work with us.

Materials and Resources

This appendix is provided for therapists who may be unfamiliar with drawing materials and resources for drawing supplies. The first section describes the two basic materials that go into drawing: paper (a surface on which to draw) and drawing tools (something with which to draw). The final section lists resources for drawing materials suitable for work with children.

PAPER

Paper comes in various sizes and types, and it is important to have at least a small assortment of papers on hand. This assortment should include good quality, white drawing paper in 8″ × 10″, 9″ × 12″, and 18″ × 24″ sheets. Colored construction paper is important to have available for children who may respond to drawing on colored backgrounds. Some therapists prefer gray paper for some drawing tasks, the rationale being that a background color other than white encourages children to use other colors, including white. White or brown Kraft paper is appropriate for murals and large individual drawing or painting projects; it generally comes in rolls 24″ or 36″ inches wide. This paper can be cut to any size, can withstand tempera and poster paint, and comes on economical rolls so the therapist can cut the sizes needed.

Most therapists use standard 8½″ × 11″ inch paper (usually copier paper), mainly because it is easy to obtain, but this is not always the best type of paper for all drawing tasks. Although materials like oil or chalk pastels (see below) can be used on simple white copier paper, these drawing materials really require a heavier grade of paper. A white paper of 60 or 80 pounds in 18″ × 24″ sheets is readily available in 100-sheet sketchbook formats, and the therapist can cut these down to make smaller sheets if the additional cost of buying other sizes is a concern. Newsprint pads are also available, but I do not recommend them for use with children; the thinness of the paper is frustrating and will not withstand any heavy coloring, shading, or pressured lines. For chalk pastels, a paper with a texture or "tooth" is best, in order to hold the pigment on paper.

DRAWING TOOLS

For some readers who are unfamiliar with art materials, the variety of drawing tools available may be as mysterious as children's drawings themselves. Many therapists rely solely on one drawing medium, such as pencils or crayons, especially if they regularly use standardized drawing assessments and evaluations with children. However, it is important to have a variety of media for drawing accessible because children's expressiveness benefits from the availability of a broad range.

A basic assortment of drawing tools for use with children should include the following: graphite pencils with good quality erasers, colored pencils, 24-color sets of crayons, felt markers (both thin and thick), and colored chalks offer a wide range of expression for children. In addition, oil pastels (also called Cray-Pas) provide the opportunity to blend colors and are also less messy than chalks. All of these drawing materials are easily transportable if the therapist is itinerant. Some drawing media can also be used as paint (e.g., Payons or water crayons) and are worth including because they offer children a medium that is more expressive than pencils or felt markers. These materials are particularly excellent for situations where "messiness" is a concern or traditional tempera or poster paints are not available.

Although many people who work with children offer thick, round-tipped crayons for drawings, this particular type of crayon may be frustrating for both young and older children to use. As children begin to make figures and add details to their drawings, small crayons will give them a less frustrating way to draw buttons, teeth, nails, fingers, and toes, and facial features that they may want to add. While the smaller crayons do break more easily than the large ones, they encourage and allow children to make more distinctions and details in their drawings. I keep both small and large crayons on hand and ask the child which is more comfortable for him or her to use; in most cases, children chose the smaller size. In any case, query the "consumer"—children will generally tell the therapist what works best for them.

When using chalks or oil pastels, the therapist may want to use a fixative (a spray preservative applied to artwork) after the drawing is completed to keep the image from smudging. Although there are a great many fixatives that artists use on their drawings to prevent smudging, a can of hairspray will do the job fairly well and will be less toxic than the commercial products. However, if you use hairspray or other fixative to fix a drawing, it should be used by the therapist and in a well-ventilated area.

RESOURCES

Many of the materials described in the previous section are available at local art or office supply stores. However, it is possible to order specific materials through the following art supply catalogues.

Triarco Arts & Crafts
14650 28th Avenue No.
Plymouth, MN 55447
800-328-3360

NASCO Arts & Crafts
901 Janesville Avenue
Fort Atkinson, WI 53538-0901
414-563-2446

Pearl Art Supplies
308 Canal Street
New York, NY 10013
800-221-6845

References

Allan, J. (1988). *Inscapes of the child's world: Jungian counseling in schools and clinics*. Dallas, TX: Spring.

Alland, A. (1983). *Playing with form: Children draw in six cultures*. New York: Columbia University Press.

Alschuler, R., & Hattwick, L. A. (1943). Easel painting as an index of personality in pre-school children. *Journal of Orthopsychiatry, 13*, 616–625.

Alschuler, R., & Hattwick, L. A. (1947). *Painting and personality: A study of young children*. Chicago: University of Chicago Press.

American Art Therapy Association (AATA). (1996). *Art therapy: Definition of the profession*. Mundelein, IL: Author.

American Art Therapy Association (AATA). (1995). *Ethical standards for art therapists*. Mundelein, IL: Author.

American Psychiatric Association. (1994). *Diagnostic and statistical manual of mental disorders* (4th ed.). Washington, DC: Author.

Anderson, F. (1992). *Art for all the children*. Springfield, IL: Charles C Thomas.

Anthony, E. J. (1986). Children's reactions to severe stress. *Journal of the American Academy of Child Psychiatry, 25*(3), 299–305.

Appel, K. (1931). Drawings by children as aids in personality studies. *American Journal of Orthopsychiatry, 1*, 129–144.

Arnheim, R. (1969). *Visual thinking*. Berkeley: University of California Press.

Arnheim, R. (1972). *Toward a psychology of art*. Berkeley: University of California Press.

Arnheim, R. (1974). *Art and visual perception*. Berkeley: University of California Press.

Arnheim, R. (1980). The puzzle of Nadia's drawings. *The Arts in Psychotherapy, 7*(2), 79–85.

Arnheim, R. (1992). *To the rescue of art*. Berkeley: University of California Press.

Axline, V. (1969). *Play therapy*. New York: Ballatine.

Bach, S. (1966). Spontaneous paintings of severely ill patients. *Acta Psychosomatica, 8*, 1–66.

Bach, S. (1975). Spontaneous pictures of leukemic children as an expression of the total personality, mind and body. *Acta Paedopsychiatrica, 41*(3), 86–104.

Bach, S. (1990). *Life paints its own span.* Einsiedeln, Switzerland: Daimon Verlag.

Banks, E. (1990).Concepts of health and sickness of pre-school and school-aged children. *Children's Health Care, 19*(1), 43–48.

Betensky, M. (1995). *What do you see?: Phenomenology of therapeutic art expression.* London: Jessica Kingsley.

Briere, J. (1992). *Child abuse trauma: Theory and treatment of the lasting effects.* Newbury Park, CA: Sage.

Buck, J. (1948). *The House–Tree–Person technique.* Los Angeles: Western Psychological Services.

Buck, J. (1966). *The House–Tree–Person technique: Revised manual.* Los Angeles: Western Psychological Services.

Burns, R. (1982). *Self-growth in families: Kinetic-Family-Drawings (K-F-D) research applications.* New York: Brunner/Mazel.

Burns, R., & Kaufman, S. H. (1972). *Actions, styles and symbols in Kinetic Family Drawings (K-F-D).* New York: Brunner/Mazel.

Burt, C. (1921). *Mental and scholastic tests.* London: P.S. King & Son.

Campanelli, M. (1991). Art therapy and ethno-cultural issues. *American Journal of Art Therapy, 30*(2), 34–35.

Cane, F. (1951). *The artist in each of us.* New York: Pantheon.

Cantlay, L.(1996). *Detecting child abuse: Recognizing children at risk through drawings.* Santa Barbara, CA: Holly Press

Case, C. & Dalley, T. (Eds.). (1990). *Working with children in art therapy.* New York: Tavistock/Routledge.

Center for Children with Chronic Illness and Disability. (1996). Factors associated with risk and resiliency. *Children's and Youths' Health Issues, 4*(1), 6–7.

Cohen, B., & Cox, C. T. (1995). *Telling without talking: Art as a window into the world of multiple personality.* New York: Norton.

Cohen, B., Hammer, J., & Singer, S. (1988). Diagnostic Drawing Series: A systematic approach to art therapy evaluation and research. *The Arts in Psychotherapy, 15,* 11–21.

Cohen, F. W., & Phelps, R. E. (1985). Incest markers in children's artwork. *The Arts in Psychotherapy, 12* 265–283.

Cohen-Liebman, M. S. (1994). The art therapist as expert witness in child sexual abuse litigation. *Art Therapy: Journal of the American Art Therapy Association, 11*(4), 260–265.

Coles, R. (1990). *The spiritual life of children.* Boston: Houghton Mifflin.

Cooke, E. (1885). *Art teaching and child nature.* London: London Journal of Education.

Corey, G., Corey, M. S., & Callanan, P. (1993). *Issues and ethics in the helping professions:* Pacific Grove, CA: Brooks/Cole.

Cox, C. T. (1984). *Themes of self-destruction: Indicators of suicidal ideation in art therapy.* Unpublished thesis, George Washington University, Washington, DC.

Cox, M. (1989). Children's drawings. In D. Hargreaves (Ed.), *Children and the arts* (pp. 43–57) Bristol, PA: Taylor & Francis.

Cox, M., & Parkin, C. (1986). Young children's human figure drawing: Cross-sectional and longitudinal studies. *Educational Psychology, 6,* 353–368.

Dennis, W. (1966). *Group values through children's drawings.* New York: Wiley.

DiLeo, J. (1970). *Young children and their drawings.* New York: Brunner/Mazel.

DiLeo, J. (1973). *Children's drawings as diagnostic aids.* New York: Brunner/Mazel.

DiLeo, J. (1983). *Interpreting children's drawings.* New York: Brunner/Mazel.

Dissanayake, E. (1989). *What is art for?* Seattle: University of Washington Press.

Drachnik, C. (1994). The tongue as a graphic symbol of sexual abuse. *Art Therapy: Journal of the American Art Therapy Association, 11*(1), 58–61.

Drachnik, C. (1995). *Interpreting metaphors in children's drawings.* Burlingame, CA: Abbeygate Press.

Epperson, J. (1990). *Environmental drawings and behaviors in children from violent homes.* Unpublished thesis, University of Utah, Salt Lake City.

Faller, K. (1988). *Child sexual abuse: New theory and research.* New York: Columbia University Press.

Field, P. A., & Morse, J. M. (1985). *Qualitative nursing research: The application of qualitative approaches.* Rockville, MD: Aspen.

Freeman, J., Epston, D., & Lobovits, D. (1997). *Playful approaches to serious problems: Narrative therapy with children and their families.* New York: Norton.

Freud, A. (1926). *The ego and mechanisms of defense.* New York: International Universities Press.

Freud, A. (1946). *Normality and pathology in childhood: Assessments of development.* New York: International Universities Press.

Furth, G. (1988). *The secret world of drawings.* Boston: Sigo Press.

Furth, G. (1981). The use of drawings made at significant times in one's life. In E. Kübler-Ross, *Living with death and dying* (pp. 63–93). New York: Macmillan.

Gantt, L. (1990). *A validity study of the Formal Elements Art Therapy Scale (FEATS) for diagnostic information in patients' drawings.* Unpublished doctoral dissertation, University of Pittsburgh, Pittsburgh, PA.

Gantt, L., & Tabone, C. (1998). *Rating scale for the Formal Elements Art Therapy Scale.* Morgantown, VA: Gargoyle Press.

Gardner, H. (1979). Children's art: Nadia's challenge. *Psychology Today, 13*(4), 18–23.

Gardner, H. (1980). *Artful scribbles: The significance of children's drawings.* New York: Basic Books.

Gardner, H. (1982). *Art, mind, and brain.* New York: Basic Books.

Gil, E. (1991). *The healing power of play.* New York: Guilford Press.

Gil, E. (1994). *Play in family therapy.* New York: Guilford Press.

Gillespie, J. (1994). *The projective use of mother-and-child drawings: A manual for clinicians.* New York: Brunner/Mazel.

Gillespie, J. (1997). Projective mother-and-child drawings. In E. Hammer

(Ed.), *Advances in projective drawing interpretation* (pp. 137–151). Springfield, IL: Charles C Thomas.

Golomb, C. (1981). Representation and reality: The origins and determinants of young children's drawings. *Review of Research in Visual Arts Education, 14*, 36–48.

Golomb, C. (1990). *The child's creation of a pictorial world.* Berkeley: University of California Press.

Goodenough, F. (1926). *Measurement of intelligence by drawings.* New York: Harcourt, Brace, & World.

Graham, J. (1994). The art of emotionally disturbed adolescents: Designing a drawing program to address violent imagery. *American Journal of Art Therapy, 32*(4), 115–121.

Green, A. (1983). The dimensions of psychological trauma in abused children. *Journal of the American Academy of Child Psychiatry, 22*, 231–237.

Gregorian, V. S., Azarian, A., DeMaria, M., & McDonald, L. D. (1996). Colors of disaster: The psychology of the "black sun." *The Arts in Psychotherapy, 23*(1), 1–14.

Gregory, P. (1990). *Body map of feelings.* Lethbridge, Alberta: Family and Community Development Program.

Gulbro-Leavitt, C., & Schimmel, B. (1991). Assessing depression in children and adolescents using the Diagnostic Drawing Series modified for children (DDS-C). *The Arts in Psychotherapy, 18*, 353–356.

Haeseler, M. (1987). Censorship or intervention: But you said we could draw whatever we wanted! *American Journal of Art Therapy, 26*(1), 11–20.

Hammer, E. (1958). *The clinical application of projective drawings.* Springfield, IL: Charles C Thomas.

Hammer, E. (1997). *Advances in projective drawing interpretation.* Springfield, IL: Charles C Thomas.

Harris, D. (1963). *Children's drawings as measures of intellectual maturity.* New York: Harcourt, Brace & World.

Henley, D. (1989). Nadia revisited: A study into the nature of regression in the autistic savant syndrome. *Art Therapy: Journal of the American Art Therapy Association, 6*(2), 43–56.

Henley, D. (1992). *Exceptional children, exceptional art: Teaching art to special needs.* Worcester, MA: Davis.

Herberholz, B., & Hanson, L. (1985). *Early childhood art* (3rd ed.). Dubuque, IA: W. C. Brown.

Herl. T. (1992). Finding the light at the end of the funnel: Working with child survivors of the Andover Tornado. *Art Therapy: Journal of the American Art Therapy Association, 9*(1), 42–47.

Hibbard, R., Roghmann, K., & Hoekelman, R. (1987). Genitalia in children's drawings: An association with sexual abuse. *Pediatrics, 79*(1), 129–137.

Hulse, W. (1952). Childhood conflict expressed through family drawings. *Journal of Projective Techniques, 16*, 66–79.

Jolles, I. (1971). *A catalogue for the qualitative interpretation of the*

House–Tree–Person (H-T-P). Los Angeles: Western Psychological Services.

Jung, C. G. (1954). *The practice of psychotherapy*. New York: Pantheon.

Jung, C. G. (1956). *The collected works. Vol. 5. Symbols of transformation*. Princeton: Princeton University Press.

Jung, C. G. (1960). *Man and his symbols*. New York: Dell.

Junge, M. B., & Asawa, P. P. (1994). *A history of art therapy in the United States*. Mundelein, IL: American Art Therapy Association.

Kashini, J. H., Husain, A., Shekin, W., Hodges, K., Cytryn, L., & McNew, D. (1981). Current perspectives on childhood depression: An overview. *American Journal of Psychiatry, 138*, 143–152.

Kellogg, J. (1993). *Mandala: Path of beauty*. Lightfoot, VA: MARI.

Kellogg, R. (1969). *Analyzing children's art*. Palo Alto, CA: Mayfield.

Kelley, S. J. (1984). The use of art therapy with sexually abused children. *Journal of Psychosocial Nursing, 22*, 12–18.

Kelley, S. J. (1985). Drawings: Critical communication for sexually abused children. *Pediatric Nursing, 11*(6), 421–426.

Knowles, L. P. (1996). Art therapists exhibiting children's art: When, where, and why. *Art Therapy: Journal of the American Art Therapy Association, 13*(3), 205–207.

Koppitz, E. (1968). *Psychological evaluation of children's human figure drawings*. New York: Grune & Stratton.

Koppitz, E. (1984). *Psychological evaluation of human figure drawings by middle school pupils*. New York: Grune & Stratton.

Kramer, E. (1993). *Art as therapy with children*. Chicago: Magnolia Street Publishers.

Kramer, E., Gerity, L., Henley, D., & Williams, K. (1995). *Art and art therapy and the seductive environment*. Paper presented at the 26th annual conference of the American Art Therapy Association. San Diego, CA.

Kübler-Ross, E. (1983). *On children and death*. New York: Macmillan.

Levick, M. (1983). *They could not talk and so they drew*. Springfield, IL: Charles C Thomas.

Levick, M. (1986). *Mommy, Daddy, look what I'm saying: What children are telling us through their drawings*. New York: Evans.

Levick, M. (1997). *See what I'm saying*. Dubuque, IA: Islewest.

Levick, M., Safran, D., & Levine, A. (1990). Art therapists as expert witnesses: A judge delivers a precedent-setting decision. *The Arts in Psychotherapy, 17*, 49–53.

Levinson, P. (1986). Identification of child abuse in the art and play products of pediatric burn patients. *Art Therapy: Journal of the American Art Therapy Association, 3*(2), 61–66.

Lewis, D. W., Middlebrook, M., Mehallick, L., Rauch, T. M., Deline, C., & Thomas, E. (1996). Pediatric headaches: What do children want? *Headache, 36*(4), 224–230.

Lindstrom, M. (1957). *Children's art: A study of normal development in children's mode of visualization*. Berkeley: University of California Press.

Lombroso, C. (1895). *The man of genius*. London: Scott.

Lowenfeld, V. (1947). *Creative and mental growth*. New York: Macmillan.

Lowenfeld, V., & Brittain, W. (1982). *Creative and mental growth* (7th ed.). New York: Macmillan.

MacGregor, J. (1989). *The discovery of the art of the insane*. Lawrenceville, NJ: Princeton University Press.

Machover, K. (1949). *Personality projection in the drawing of the human figure*. Springfield, IL: Charles C Thomas.

Malchiodi, C. (1982). *Your journal for growth and discovery*. Salt Lake City, UT: Women in Jeopardy Program.

Malchiodi, C. (1990). *Breaking the silence: Art therapy with children from violent homes*. New York: Brunner/Mazel.

Malchiodi, C. (1993). Medical art therapy: Contributions to the field of arts medicine. *International Journal of Arts Medicine, 2*(2), 28–31.

Malchiodi, C. (1994). Writing about art therapy for professional publication. *Art Therapy: Journal of the American Art Therapy Association, 9*(2), 62–64.

Malchiodi, C. (1996). Documentation and case presentations. In C. Malchiodi & S. Riley, *Supervision and related issues* (pp. 155–175). Chicago: Magnolia Street Publishers.

Malchiodi, C. (1997). *Breaking the silence: Art therapy with children from violent homes* (2nd ed., rev.). New York: Brunner/Mazel.

Malchiodi, C., & Riley, S. (1996). *Supervision and related issues*. Chicago: Magnolia Street Publishers.

Martin, R. (1988). Ethics column. *School Psychologist, 8,* 5–8.

Matorana, A. (1954). *A comparison of the personal, emotional, and family adjustments of crippled and normal children*. Unpublished doctoral thesis, University of Minnesota, Minneapolis, MN.

Miller, A. (1986). *Pictures of a childhood*. New York: Farrar, Straus, & Giroux.

Mitchell, J., & McArthur, R. (1994). *Human Figure Drawing Test (HFDT): An illustrated handbook for clinical interpretation and standardized assessment of cognitive impairment*. Los Angeles: Western Psychological Services.

Morris, D. (1962). *The biology of art*. London: Methuen.

Moustakas, C. (1959). *Psychotherapy with children*. New York: Harper.

Naumburg, M. (1973). *An introduction to art therapy: Studies of "free" art expression of behavior problem children and adolescents as means of diagnosis and therapy*. New York: Teachers College Press. (Original work published 1947)

Naumburg, M. (1987). *Dynamically oriented art therapy: Its principles and practice*. Chicago: Magnolia Street Publishers. (Original work published 1966)

Neale, E.L. (1994). The children's diagnostic drawing series. *Art Therapy: Journal of the American Art Therapy Association, 11*(2), 119–126.

Oaklander, V. (1978). *Windows to our children*. Moab, UT: Real People Press.

Oster, G., & Gould, P. (1987). *Using drawings in assessment and therapy*. New York: Brunner/Mazel.

Oster, G., & Montgomery, S. (1996). *Clinical uses of drawings.* Northvale, NJ: Jason Aronson.

Ounsted, C., Oppenheimer, R. and Lindsay, J. (1974). Aspects of bonding failure: The psychotherapeutic treatment of families of battered children. *Developmental Medicine and Child Neurology, 16,* 446–456.

Pasto, T. (1965). *The space–frame experience in art.* New York: A. S. Barnes & Co.

Perkins, C. (1977). The art of life-threatened children: A preliminary study. In R. Shoemaker & S. Gonick-Barris (Eds.), *Creativity and the art therapist's identity: The proceedings of the Seventh Annual Conference of the American Art Therapy Association* (pp. 9–12). Baltimore: American Art Therapy Association.

Pfeffer, C. (1986). *The suicidal child.* New York: Guilford Press.

Piaget, J. (1959). *Judgment and reasoning in the child.* Patterson, NJ: Littlefield, Adams.

Piaget, J., & Inhelder, B. (1971). *Mental imagery in the child.* New York: Basic Books.

Pinderhughes, E. (1989). *Understanding race, ethnicity, and power.* New York: Free Press.

Prinzhorn, H. (1972). *Artistry of the mentally ill.* New York: Springer.

Putnam, F. (1989). *Diagnosis and treatment of multiple personality disorder.* New York: Guilford Press.

Putnam, F., Guroff, J., Silberman, E., Barban, L., & Post, R. (1986). The clinical phenomenology of multiple personality disorder: Review of 100 recent cases. *Journal of Clinical Psychiatry, 47*(6), 285–293.

Pynoos, R., & Eth, S. (1985). Developmental perspective on psychic trauma in childhood. In C. R. Figley (Ed.), *Trauma and its wake: The study and treatment of post-traumatic stress disorder* (pp. 193–216). New York: Brunner/Mazel.

Rak, C., & Patterson, L. (1996). Promoting resilience in at-risk children. *Journal of Counseling and Development, 74*(4), 368–373.

Ricci, C. (1887). *The art of children.* Bologna, Italy.

Riley, S. (1997). Children's art and narratives: An opportunity to enhance therapy and a supervisory challenge. *The Supervision Bulletin, 9*(3), 2–3.

Roeback, H. (1968). Human figure drawings: Their utility in the psychologist's armamentarium for personality assessment. *Psychological Bulletin, 70*(1), 1–19.

Roje, J. (1995). LA '94 earthquake in the eyes of children: Art therapy with elementary school children who were victims of disaster. *Art Therapy: Journal of the American Art Therapy Association, 12*(4), 237–243.

Rubin, J. (1984a). *Child art therapy* (2nd ed.). New York: Van Nostrand Reinhold.

Rubin, J. (1984b). *The art of art therapy.* New York: Brunner/Mazel.

Saint Exupéry, A. de (1943). *The little prince.* New York: Harcourt Brace Jovanovich.

Selfe, L. (1977). *Nadia: A case of extraordinary drawing ability in an autistic child.* New York: Academic Press.

Shoemaker, R. (1984). *The rainbow booklet*. Baltimore: Renewing Visions Press.

Silver, R. (1978). *Developing cognitive and creative skills through art*. Baltimore: University Park Press.

Silver, R. (1988). *Draw a story*. New York: Ablin Press.

Silver, R. (1993). *Draw a story* (rev. ed.). New York: Ablin Press.

Silver, R. (1996a). *Silver Drawing Test of cognition and emotion*. Sarasota, FL: Ablin Press.

Silver, R. (1996b). Sex differences in the solitary and assaultive fantasies of delinquent and nondelinquent adolescents. *Adolescence, 31*(123), 543–552.

Silver, R. (1997). Sex and age differences in attitudes toward the opposite sex. *Art Therapy: Journal of the American Art Therapy Association, 14*(4), 286–272.

Silvern, L., Karyl, J., & Landis, T. (1995). Individual psychotherapy for traumatized children of abused women. In E. Peled, P. Jaffe, & L. Edleson (Eds.), *Ending the cycle of violence* (pp. 43–76). Thousand Oaks, CA: Sage.

Simon, M. (1876). L'imagination dans la folie. *Annale Médico-Psychologie, 16*, 358–390.

Sobol, B., & Cox, C.T. (Speakers). (1992). *Art and dissociation: Research with sexually abused children* (Cassette recording #59–144). Denver: National Audio Video.

Steele, B. (1997). *Trauma response kit: Short term intervention model*. Grosse Pointe Woods, MI: Institute for Trauma and Loss in Children.

Steele, B., Ginns-Gruenberg, D., & Lemerand, P. (1995). *I feel better now!: Leader's guide*. Grosse Pointe Woods, MI: Institute for Trauma and Loss in Children.

Stronach-Bushel, B. (1990). Trauma, children and art. *American Journal of Art Therapy, 29*, 48– 52.

Swenson, E. (1968). Empirical evaluations of human figure drawings; 1957–1966. *Psychological Bulletin, 70*(1), 20–44.

Tardieu, L. (1872). *Etude médico-légale sur la folie*. Paris: Baillière.

Terr, L. (1981). Forbidden games: Post-traumatic child's play. *Journal of the American Academy of Child Psychiatry, 20*, 741–760.

Terr, L. (1990). *Too scared to cry*. New York: Basic Books.

Tibbetts, T. (1989). Characteristics of artwork in children with post-traumatic stress disorder in Northern Ireland. *Art Therapy: Journal of the American Art Therapy Association, 6*(3), 92–98.

Toll, N. (1993). *Behind the secret window: A memoir of a hidden childhood during World War II*. New York: Dial.

Uhlin, D. (1979). *Art for exceptional children*. Dubuque, IA: William Brown.

Wadeson, H. (1971). Characteristics of art expression in depression. *Journal of Nervous and Mental Disease, 153*(3), 197–204.

Wass, H. (1984). Concepts of death: A developmental perspective. In H. Wass & C. Corr (Eds.), *Childhood and death* (pp. 3–23). Washington, DC: Hemisphere.

Webb, N. B. (1991). Play therapy crisis intervention with children. In N. B. Webb (Ed.), *Play therapy with children in crisis* (pp. 26–42). New York: Guilford Press.

Weber, J., Cooper, K., & Hesser, J. (1996). Children's drawings of the elderly: Young ideas abandon old age stereotypes. *Art Therapy: Journal of the American Art Therapy Association, 13*(2),114–117.

Werner, E. (1992). The children of Kauai: Resiliency and recovery in adolescence and adulthood. *Journal of Adolescent Health, 13,* 262–268.

White, M., & Epston, D. (1990). *Narrative means to therapeutic ends.* New York: Norton.

Wilber, K. (1996). How big is our umbrella? *Noetic Sciences Review, 40,* 10–17.

Willats, J. (1977). How children learn to represent three-dimensional space in drawings. In G. Butterworth (Ed.), *The child's representation of the world* (pp. 367–382). New York: Plenum.

Wilson, L. (1987). Confidentiality in art therapy: An ethical dilemma. *American Journal of Art Therapy, 25,* 75–80.

Winner, E. (1982). *Invented worlds: The psychology of the arts.* Cambridge, MA: Harvard University.

Winner, E. (1986, August). Where pelicans kiss seals. *Psychology Today,* pp. 25–35.

Winnicott, D. (1971). *Playing and reality.* New York: Basic Books.

Wolff, W. (1942). Projective methods for personality analysis of expressive behavior in pre-school children. *Character and Personality, 10,* 309–330.

Wohl, A., & Kaufman, B. (1985). *Silent screams and hidden cries: An interpretation of artwork by children from violent homes.* New York: Brunner/Mazel.

Yates, A., Buetler, L. E., & Crago, M. (1985). Drawings by child victims of incest. *Child Abuse and Neglect: An International Journal, 9*(2), 183–190.

Index